Healthy Back Building

Healthy Back Building

Tips and Exercises to Prevent Back Pain

WILLIAM WHITNEY, D.C., M.A.

FOREWORD BY
AUBREY SWARTZ, M.D.

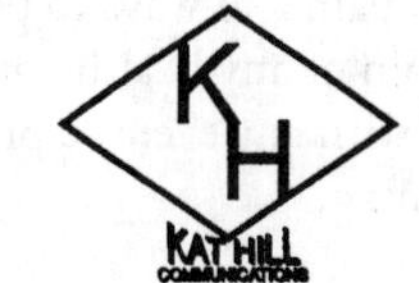

KAT HILL PRESS
an imprint of

KAT HILL COMMUNICATIONS
ANTIOCH, CALIFORNIA

Healthy Back Building, by William Whitney, DC, MA. Printed and bound in the United States of America. **All rights reserved**. No part of this book may be reproduced in any form or by any electronic or mechanical means including information storage and retrieval systems without permission in writing from the author, except by a reviewer, who may quote brief passages in a review. Published by Kat Hill Press, an imprint of Kat Hill Communications, PO Box 3044, Antioch, California 94531. E-mail: kathill@ccnet.com. First edition, July 1997.

Publisher's - Cataloging-in-Publication Data
(Prepared by Quality Books Inc.)
Whitney, William, 1958-
Healthy back building : tips and exercises to prevent back pain / William Whitney ; foreword by Aubrey Swartz.
p. cm.
Includes bibliographical references and index.
1. Backache—Exercise therapy. 2. Health promotion. 3. Back-care and hygiene. 4. Backache prevention. I. Title.
Preassigned LCCN: 96-77524
ISBN: 0-9654729-4-9
RD771.B217W45 1997 617.5′64
QB196-40666

Typesetting and cover design by Joel Friedlander

Disclaimer: The information in this book was not intended for the treatment of back pain. It is intended to provide a framework about understanding the risk of back pain and ways to possibly lower one's risk. If you suffer from back pain or any health condition seek the care of your doctor. In addition, as with any exercise program always consult with your doctor before beginning.

The following page is an extension of this copyright page.

PERMISSIONS

Excerpts from *Bicycling Magazine*: Copyright by BICYCLING magazine. Reproduced by permission. For subscription information, call 1-800-666-2806.

"Calories Burned during Tour de France:," which appeared in Paceline by Bill Strickland (8/92, PG. 16)

Statements "Taking it when sitting and standing and noting the Difference. Lie back down. The normal difference is 3-5 beats. Hard training. 5-8 beats." Which appear in Coach Approach, Eddie B., by Geoff Drake (4/92, PG. 82)

Excerpts from the American College of Sports Medicine's *Guidelines for Exercise Testing and Prescription*. Hamstring flexibility and rate of progression of exercise. Copyright Williams & Wilkins. Reproduced by permission.

Written by the American College of Sports Medicine, Guidelines for Exercise Testing and Prescription, 4th edition, Williams & Wilkins, 1991, PG. 107-11.

Excerpts from "International Society of Sports Psychology Position Statement: Physical Activity and Psychological Benefits." Copyright by International Society of Sports Psychology. Permission to reproduce material granted by ISSP's Permissions Department, School of Sport Psychology, University of Southern Queensland, Toowoomba, Queensland, Australia 4350.

Excerpts from the *Journal of The American Dietetic Association*," statement position, July 1987. Copyright The American Dietetic Association. Reprinted by permission from JOURNAL OF THE AMERICAN DIETETIC ASSOCIATION, Vol. 87: PG. 935-7.

Excerpts from *Manipulative Therapy in Rehabilitation of the Motor System*, 2nd edition, by Karel Lewit. "Muscle groups that show a tendency to hyperactivity or inhibition, Table 2.1, PG. 32." Copyright by Butterworths-Heinemann Ltd.: Oxford England. Reproduced by permission.

Excerpts from *Medicine and Science in Sports and Exercise*. Table describing Borg Scale, by Gunner Borg. Copyright Williams & Wilkins. Reproduced by permission.

Borg, G.A.V., "Psychophysical Bases of Perceived Exertion." MEDICINE AND SCIENCE IN SPORTS AND EXERCISE, Vol. 14, 5: PG. 378.

Excerpts from *The New England Journal of Medicine*, regarding disc abnormalities in healthy individuals by Maureen C. Jensen, et al. Reproduced by permission.

Excerpted with permission from THE NEW ENGLAND JOURNAL OF MEDICINE; M.C. Jensen, et al., "Magnetic Resonance Imaging Of The Lumbar Spine In People Without Back Pain," Vol. 331, 2: PG. 70-2, 1994. Copyright 1991. Massachusetts Medical Society. All rights reserved.

Excerpts from *NSCA Journal/Strength & Conditioning*. Copyright National Strength & Conditioning Association. Reproduced by permission.

Wathen, D. NSCA Journal (1987) 9(5):26

"Flexibility: Its Place in Warm-up Activities."

Excerpts from *STATISTICAL BULLETIN*, Metropolitan Life Insurance, Vol. 64 Jan-June: PG. 2. Height and weight chart. Copyright by Metropolitan Life Insurance. Reproduce by permission courtesy of Metropolitan Life Insurance.

Here's what reviewers had to say:

"Back pain is at epidemic proportions and the cost to industry and quality of life is staggering. Each of us is at risk. It is for this reason that we should understand and practice the principles that are expertly presented in Dr. Whitney's outstanding book *Healthy Back Building.* The words to describe it are well organized, comprehensive, easily understood and well researched. The readers have the opportunity to understand the problem, assess their own risk and apply the principles of back building as Dr. Whitney takes them through his enjoyable back building system. The well-done illustrations, everyday examples and charts help individuals quickly and easily plan the exercises and movements that are best for their backs.

I highly recommend this unique book to anyone, especially to those wishing to build and maintain healthy backs."

Robert Boyce, Ph.D.
Exercise Physiologist
Preventive and Rehabilitation Exercise Program Director
Founder and Past Director of the Occupational Physiology Forum, American College of Sports Medicine

"**TERRIFIC!!** It is accurate and well written, but it also is extremely readable...As a biomechanist, I found the exercises to be appropriate as well as safe. And I especially like the fact that you emphasized exercising the whole body, not just specific exercises for the back."

Gail G. Evans, Ph.D.
Professor in Human Performance
San Jose State University
Past Secretary, National Association for Physical Education in Higher Education

"I would recommend this book to everyone.....Dr. Whitney introduces a safe and simple program that virtually guarantees a healthy back for a lifetime. ...each person can easily determine what he or she is doing on a regular basis that may be potentially harmful to his or her back.

This book offers the most complete spinal health care program available today."

Terry Schroeder, D.C.
Four-time Olympic athlete
Pepperdine University, Water Polo Coach

"...An excellent tool in educating the public and our patients. The most extensive material I have ever seen on... prevention of back problems in layman's terms. I can honestly say that if an individual reads this material and follows your recommendations, it will go a long way to preventing low back conditions. Considering 8 out of 10 people will suffer debilitating back conditions sometime in their life. If this material can be absorbed by the general public, they will do much to prevent such occurrences and re-occurrences. At a time when patients will soon be paying more for their health care, this type of material will save many people considerable time, money and distress. I applaud you in efforts.

This book would also benefit the general practitioners and chiropractic physicians. There are tidbits I will begin employing within my own practice. I believe every physician should review this type of material and encourage their patients to become more self educated on this topic."

Robert E. Monokian, D.C., D.A.C.B.S.P.
President of the American Chiropractic Association's, Council on Sport Injuries and Physical Fitness (1996)

"Dr. Whitney is commended on the excellent job he has done in developing a comprehensive publication which combines a practical, common-sense and clinical approach which is scientifically valid...."

Aubrey Swartz, M.D.
Orthopaedic Surgeon
Executive Director, American Back Society

Acknowledgments

FIRST, I WISH TO ACKNOWLEDGE my family, the most important entity in my life. Jennifer, who's been my wife for over a decade, gave me unlimited encouragement to produce this book. I want to express my appreciation also to my daughters Kate and Hilary for their support and to my father, Gilbert Whitney, who tolerated my love for physical activity yet encouraged and supported my academic growth.

A special thanks to Mari Upton for her excellent line drawings; Sally Siino and Bill Wristen for modeling for most of the illustrations; Deborah Cady for her copyediting skills; JoAnn and Dave Hobbs for their endless proofreading and computer coaching; and my office manager, Peggy Morrow, for keeping the office running in a normal fashion while I was reviewing the biomedical literature and writing the book.

Additional thanks go to the library staffs at Diablo Valley College, Palmer College of Chiropractic (Davenport) and the University of California Medical School in San Francisco — a diligent crew who were always willing to lend a hand. How blessed I was during my writing to be surrounded by the excellent staff within the Physical Education Department at Diablo Valley College who, I might add, were always willing to answer my questions.

Thanks also to Dr. Swartz for taking the time to write the foreword for the book; Drs. Boyce, Evans, Monokian and Schroeder for their kind words; and Dr. Joseph Sweere of Northwestern College of Chiropractic, possibly the most professional and cordial person in all of the chiropractic profession, for taking time to critique the manuscript.

This book is dedicated to all those who believe in promoting good health.

Contents

Illustrations

Tables

Foreword

THIS BOOK PRESENTS a timely and well-organized program to improve the fitness, conditioning and muscular strength of the back. The health care community has accepted the concept of the adverse effects of inactivity on the disc unit, joint function, and ligamentous, tendinous and muscular tissue. There is also current acceptance of the favorable effect of aerobic exercise on these tissues in the prevention of many types of low back problems. There has been a steady trend over the past several years in back care to emphasize the role of active therapy in the form of exercise, of various types, in the prevention and the treatment of mechanical low back pain.

Dr. Whitney has organized the material presented in this book in a thoughtful, comprehensive and logical manner. This book is written in a matter that is easy to understand and that provides the reader with a basic framework upon which to build a home-conditioning program. A regular program such as this can improve neuromotor control, coordination, mechanical efficiency, and therefore can reduce the likelihood of back injury or recurrence of back pain.

Stretching exercises have been demonstrated to improve spine mobility and to help muscles and ligaments to become more limber, and especially those which have been restricted because of a painful process. The clinician is encouraged to monitor patients who are engaged in home-exercise programs in order to maximize efficacy through motivation and compliance by the patient.

Dr. Whitney has emphasized the importance of educating our patients. It is important for the clinician prescribing a home-exercise program to ensure that patients receive specific and appropriate information regarding special areas to emphasize in their own particular programs.

Dr. Whitney is commended on the excellent job he has done in developing a comprehensive publication which combines a practical, common-sense and clinical approach which is scientifically valid and current with the present state of the art.

Aubrey, A. Swartz, MD., Pharm.D.
Executive Director, American Back Society

Introduction

IF YOU HAVE EVER SUFFERED from back pain and would like to prevent it from recurring or have witnessed the effects of a backache or back disability in others and hope to prolong your own good health, this book is for you!

Other books will show you the proper way to lift, sit, sleep, and stand or advise you on what to do once you've developed pain. Unfortunately, the approaches in such books do not present ways to prevent problems in every category of the known risk factors of back pain.

This book is your complete guide to reducing the risk of back pain. It includes a number of back-building tips that will eliminate or minimize such risks and thus help you to remain healthy. This book is unique because it emphasizes exercise as a primary means to reducing your risk of developing back problems. Based on the scientific literature, this book contains the only exercise program that can have an effect on each risk category related to back pain, thus making the back-friendly workout the single most comprehensive approach you can use to prevent back problems.

Since this exercise program can also reduce your risk for cardiovascular and psychological conditions, you'll see how it is the best fitness program for promoting your overall health. In addition, you'll learn how easy it is to apply this workout and other back-building tips to your daily lifestyle and stay motivated.

CHAPTER 1

The Back-Friendly Workout

WHEN MOST PEOPLE THINK of exercising for their health, they think of how to improve their heart, reduce their waistline, or relieve emotional stress. Rarely do they give any thought to the back. Yet back pain is a leading cause of disability and the second most common reason why people visit a physician (second after the common cold). A permanent and severe back disability can result in living in constant pain. Also, once such a disability develops, it can no longer be cured.

Exercise helps to prevent back pain and lets the back work more efficiently. Many have mistakenly equated being pain-free with being healthy. It is now known that maintenance of a healthy back and body includes exercise that is performed properly and regularly.

The ideal situation when developing an exercise program is to encompass the entire body without over or underdeveloping any one area of the body (Fig. 1-1). The body needs to be treated as a single unit, and for maximum fitness, the whole body has to be developed. For example, without strong arms and legs, a person is more likely to strain his or her back when lifting. Being overweight can place exces-

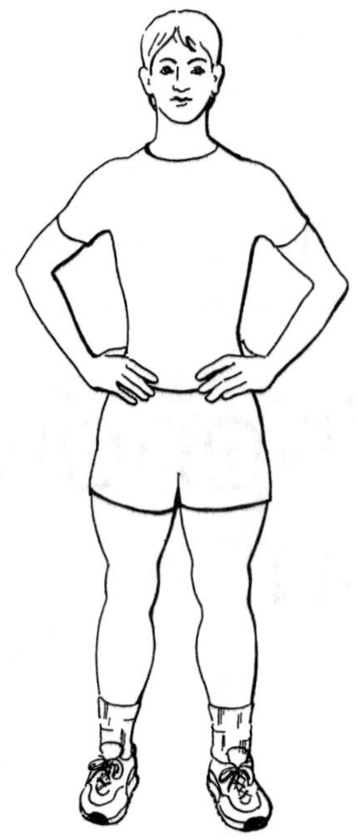

Fig. 1-1a. Lower body workout only

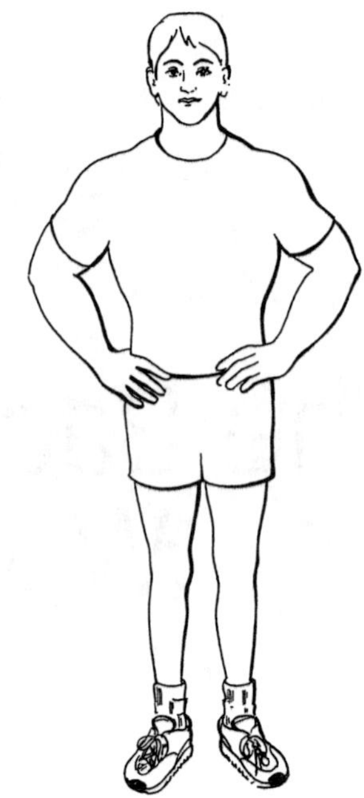

Fig. 1-1b. Upper body workout only

sive stress upon the lower back. Therefore, having a fit back really means having a fit body.

A fitness program that promotes good health involves activities that contribute to the development and maintenance of cardiovascular conditioning, flexibility, muscle strength, and muscle endurance. This means first developing an adequate level of each component and thereafter maintaining at least a minimum level in each component.

A good fitness program can be carried out in just minutes a day. One of the great aspects of exercise is that those who need it the most are the people who will get the most improvement in the shortest period of time. Unlike competitive training, this health-related fitness program involves a moderate level of training. This program also allows some variation in exercises, which prevents one from getting bored by repeating the same thing over and over.

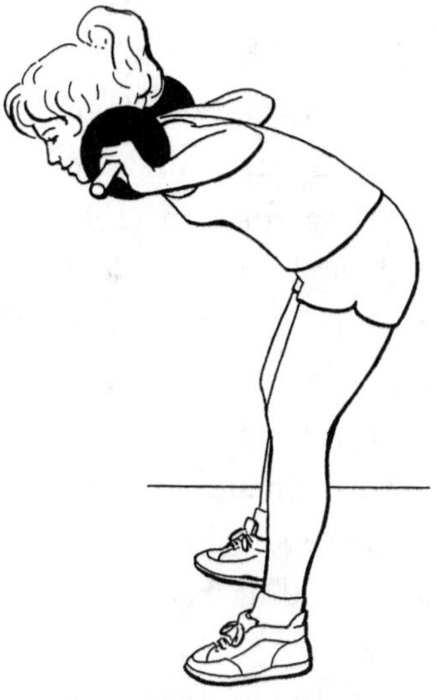

Fig. 1-2. Forward bending

The details of each fitness component are discussed later, but first, it's important to remind yourself that your goal is to achieve good health. The last thing you want is to create an injury. This is especially true of your back. Experts agree that most back pain is usually caused not by a single injury but by an accumulation of injuries. One day a person will bend over to pick up a pencil and won't be able to straighten up. Years of exposure to certain risk factors (see Chapter 3) have finally caught up with the person, and the pencil is "the straw that broke the camel's back." The accumulation of risks over time causes wear and tear to the back that eventually leads to a painful condition. In the average individual, this degenerating process typically begins to become painful at approximately 35 years of age. Low-back pain is so common at this time in life that it has been determined to be the single most expensive health care problem in the United States in the 35-55 age group.

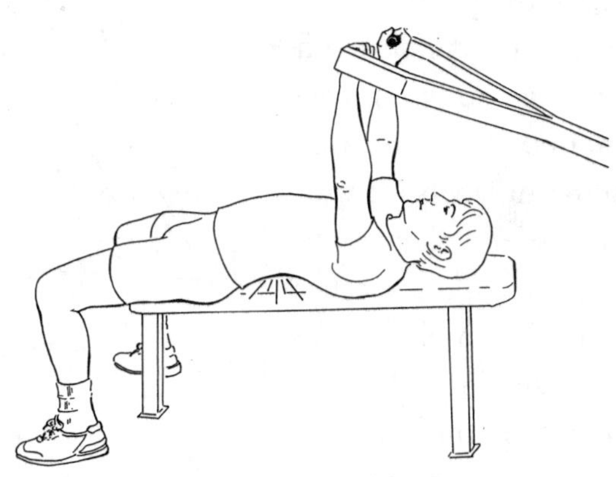

Fig. 1-3. Arching of the low back

Certain body movements have been shown to play a role in this back-degenerating process. You want to eliminate these body movements from your exercise program, since you will be working out regularly. Otherwise, your workout could put your healthy back at risk for back injury and pain.

Improper back movements include bending forward (Fig. 1-2), arching of the low back (Fig. 1-3), twisting (Fig. 1-4), carrying or reaching for loads away from and in front of the body (Fig. 1-5), and bending backward (Fig. 1-6). Avoiding these movements may seem quite restricting, but this book includes a step-by-step plan that shows you how simple it is to eliminate or minimize these improper movements.

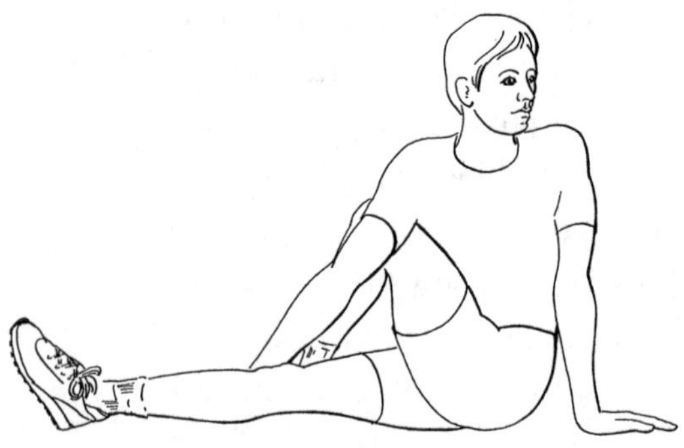

Fig. 1-4. Twisting

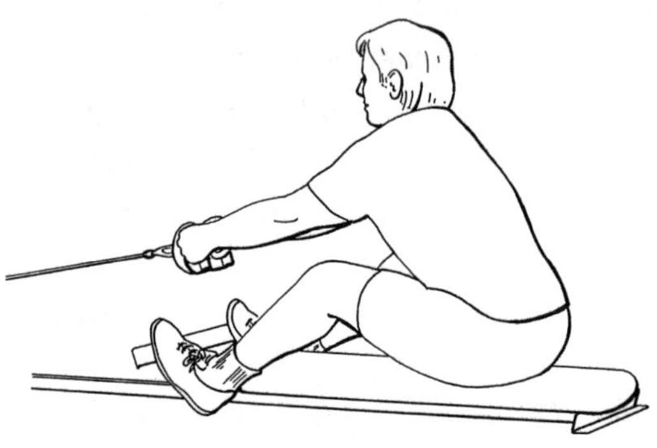

Fig. 1-5. Reaching away from body

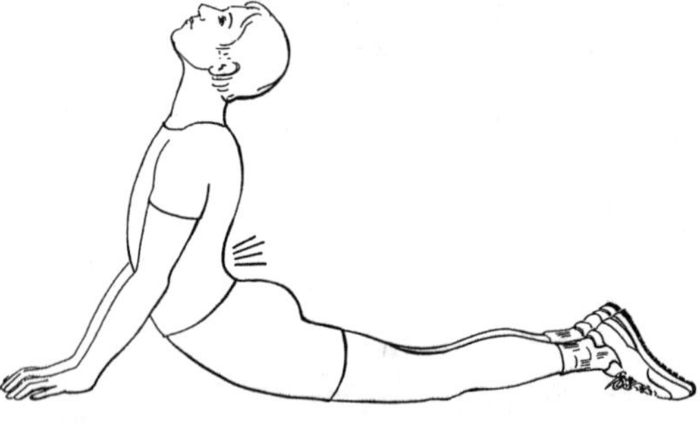

Fig. 1-6. Backward bending

A few general rules on posture will help you to understand proper body movements. The normal spine has two forward curves—one located in the neck and the other in the low back (Fig. 1-7). Our desire is to maintain these curves in our spine as much as possible during exercise. The recommended techniques used in this book for stretching, weight training, and conditioning have some movements and positions that do slightly compromise these curves. However, it's believed that the benefit of the exercise will outweigh any risk to your back. Remember that it is important at all times to concentrate on your body position and movements when working out. If you're not sure about any position, double check with this book or consult with a fitness instructor.

As a collegiate physical education instructor, I'm surprised at how few people participate in all components of exercise, especially since these components have been taught by health and physical educators for years. Yet, even today it's not hard to find the individual who simply lifts weights and does nothing else or the long-distance runner who is highly conditioned but doesn't work to increase his or her muscle strength, muscle endurance, or flexibility. These people are not completely physically fit, even though some may spend hours a day exercising.

As a practicing chiropractor, I see another common problem with individuals who exercise. On Monday morning, the weekend athlete comes into the office complaining of back pain, usually as a result of overexertion or improper repetitive body movements used while exercising.

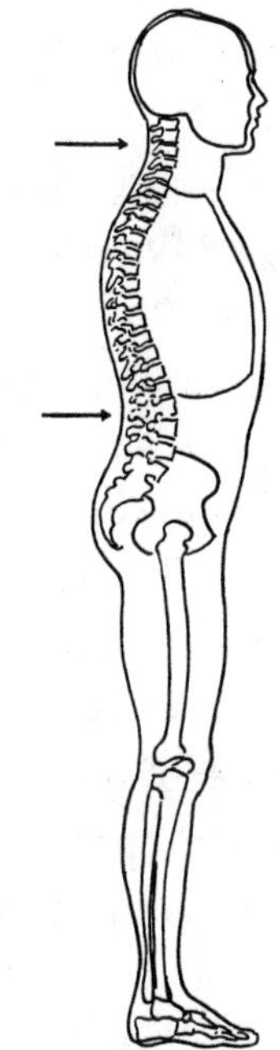

Fig. 1-7. Normal curves of the spine

The back-friendly workout provides a balance of the fitness components while eliminating the blatant improper movements related to the spine. It also emphasizes that exercise needs to be done at a moderate, and not a vigorous, level. This is helpful in reducing injuries caused by overexertion and in maintaining a workout routine. Another feature of the back-friendly workout is that your body will become active, which is necessary in reducing the many risk factors of back pain. I will show you how the back-friendly workout is the ONLY back-saving approach that minimizes (if not eliminates) each known risk category of back pain, making it the most comprehensive preventive tool to use against the development of back pain.

Of course, the back-friendly workout will benefit your general health and not just your back. Physical activity has been associated with the prevention and control of numerous health conditions, such as heart disease, high blood pressure, a certain type of diabetes, brittle bone disease, obesity, and some mental health problems. Research has also suggested that regular exercise not only will help increase your lifespan but also will help you to become more independent later in life.

The back-friendly workout comprises three components: stretching, conditioning, and weight training. Each component has a different effect on your health and is necessary to become physically fit.

In any exercise program, it is important to warm up before you exercise and cool down afterwards. Warming up is accomplished in two ways. Stretching exercises must be done before all conditioning and weight lifting. A warm-up routine should also include low-intensity movements similar to the activity that you are performing during your conditioning or weight-training workout. This means that if your conditioning workout consists of walking, you should warm up with an easy walk and then proceed to stretching before beginning your walking workout.

When recovering from exercise, it is important to continue exercising at a low level before reaching a resting state. After weight training, this is accomplished by stretching. During conditioning recovery, your cool-down should begin with low-intensity movements that will allow proper circulation to return. During exercise, the majority of bloodflow goes to your muscles, unlike the normal pattern of circulation. These low-intensity conditioning movements should last for approximately five to ten minutes, or until your heart rate is below 100 beats per minute. Then proceed with the second phase of your cool-down—stretching.

The stretching and weight-training components of the back-friendly workout follow a set routine designed to place minimal stress upon the back, while the conditioning component of this workout allows for a variety of activities. Table 1-1 presents a suggested routine that includes all three components of the back-friendly workout. This routine is for the fit individual who wishes to maintain a minimum level of fitness in the least amount of time.

TABLE 1-1

SUGGESTED BACK-FRIENDLY WORKOUT ROUTINE

Monday	Stretching warm-up 15 min.	Weight training (lower body) 20 min.	Stretching cool-down 5-10 min.
Tuesday	Rest		
Wednesday	Stretching warm-up 15 min.	Conditioning 20 min.	Stretching cool-down 5-10 min.
Thursday	Stretching warm-up 15 min.	Weight training (upper body) 20 min.	Stretching cool-down 5-10 min.
Friday	Stretching warm-up 15 min.	Conditioning 20 min.	Stretching cool-down 5-10 min.
Saturday	Rest		
Sunday	Stretching warm-up 15 min.	Conditioning 20 min.	Stretching cool-down 5-10 min.

It is best to exercise with others. Exercising with friends or family can make it fun and motivating. Also, by having a workout partner, you're able to have someone observe you to assure that you're using the proper technique in each part of your workout. This is especially the case during your weight-training routine, where a spotter can help you to maintain your safety when lifting.

A qualified fitness instructor at your local gym can demonstrate proper use of equipment and facilities, answer questions regarding physical fitness, and provide safety and emergency procedures when needed. A safe bet in finding a qualified fitness instructor is to go to a community college, where each instructor has an advanced degree in physical education. This may not be the case, however, in health clubs. It's best to find a fitness instructor at your club who is certified by the American College of Sports Medicine. Even if you have a workout partner with experience, it is still best to have a fitness expert present while exercising. If you don't have a workout partner, going to a club or school is a good way to find one. Such an environment can also provide social interaction, which can help to keep you motivated.

It is important to remember that this book is designed to educate you about your back and to improve back fitness. It is not the intent of this workout to provide rehabilitation or to relieve a back injury. As with any exercise program, always consult with your doctor before you begin.

CHAPTER 2

The Spine

BEFORE DISCUSSING THE RISK FACTORS for back pain, we want to emphasize the importance of understanding the structure of the back. The spine (Fig. 2-1) gives the back and neck structure to protect the nervous tissue and permit movement. The nervous tissue within the spine consists of the spinal cord and nerve roots. These nerve roots turn into nerves, which are distributed throughout the body (Fig. 2-2).

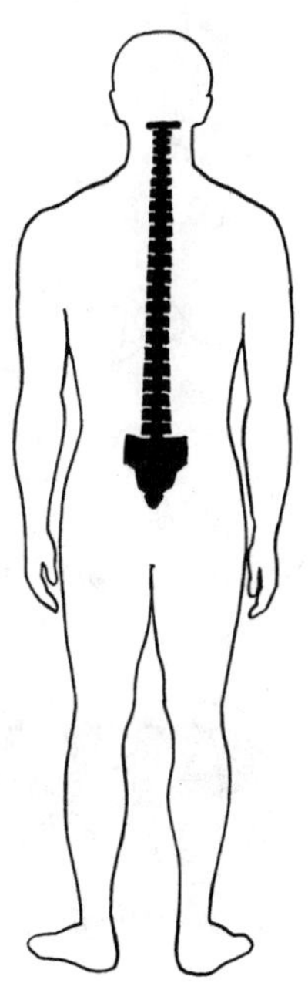

Fig. 2-1. The Spine

The spine is composed of a series of bones called vertebrae, the sacrum, and the tailbone (Fig. 2-3). Collectively, these bones are called the spinal column. There are seven vertebrae in the neck, twelve in the mid-back, and five in the low-back region. Underneath the low-back region is a bone with five fused vertebrae, called the sacrum. At the bottom of the sacrum is another bone with three to four fused vertebrae, commonly called the tailbone. The ribs attach to the sides of the mid-back

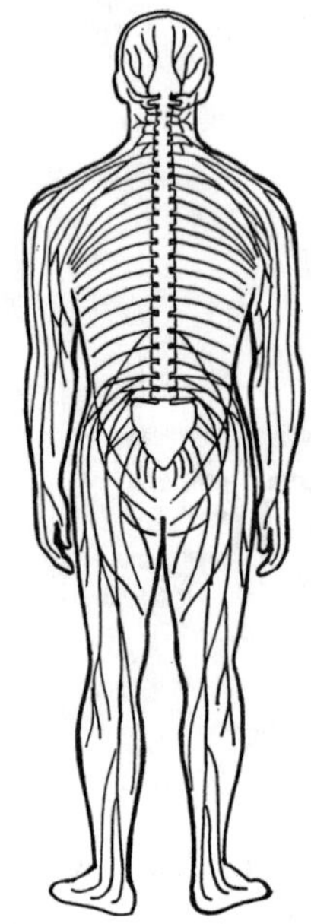

Fig. 2-2. Nerve distribution

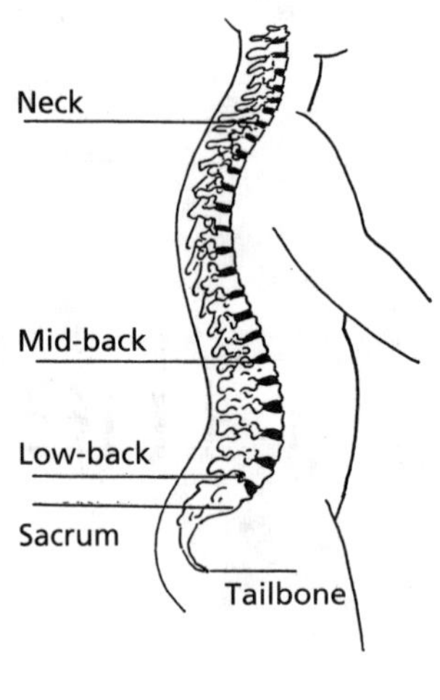

Fig. 2-3. Spinal bones

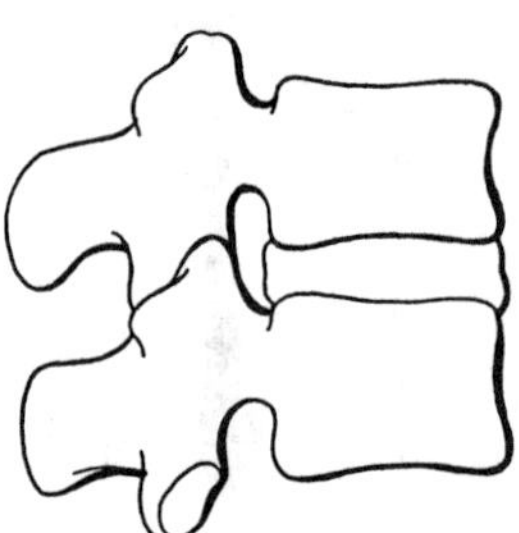

Fig. 2-4. Location of a disc

vertebrae, while the pelvis attaches to the sides of the sacrum.

Located between the vertebrae in the neck, mid-back, and low back are the discs (Fig. 2-4). An individual disc consists of two parts, the inner core and outer boundary (Fig. 2-5). The inner core is made of a jellylike substance that contains mainly water. The water content decreases with age, which is one of the reasons why adults tend to shrink in height as they grow older. The outer boundary of the disc consists of two different layers of tough elastic bands. If these elastic bands break and the jellylike substance protrudes, the condition is called a herniated disc. When the spine is compressed, a certain pres-

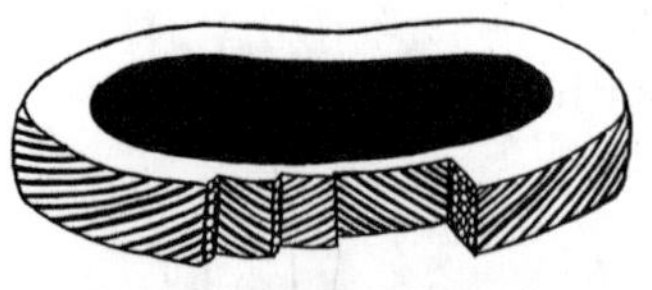

Fig. 2-5. Design of the disc

sure develops in the inner core of the disc (Fig. 2-6). This fluid pressure eventually pushes the top and bottom vertebrae away from each other. The disc thus acts as a shock absorber and transmits loads through the spine by compressing and then springing back to its normal shape.

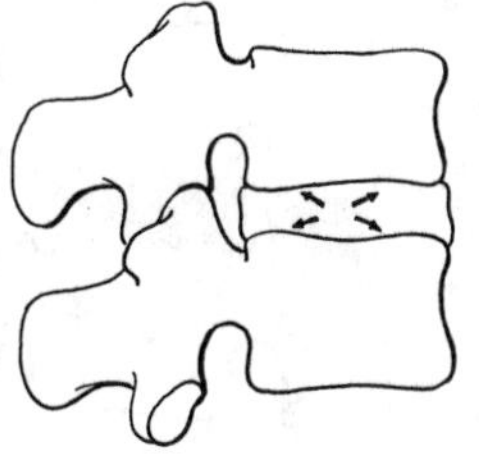

Fig. 2-6. A compressed disc

As mentioned in Chapter 1, a normal spine has two forward curves, one located in the neck and the other in the low back (Fig. 2-7). These curves give the spine both increased flexibility and shock-absorbing capacity.

The spine is supported by seven ligaments (Fig 2-8). Like a disc, a ligament connects bone to bone. The ligaments help the spine work in several ways: they can absorb large loads applied to the spine, allow smooth motion, help maintain posture with a minimum of energy, and restrict motion to stay within normal limits.

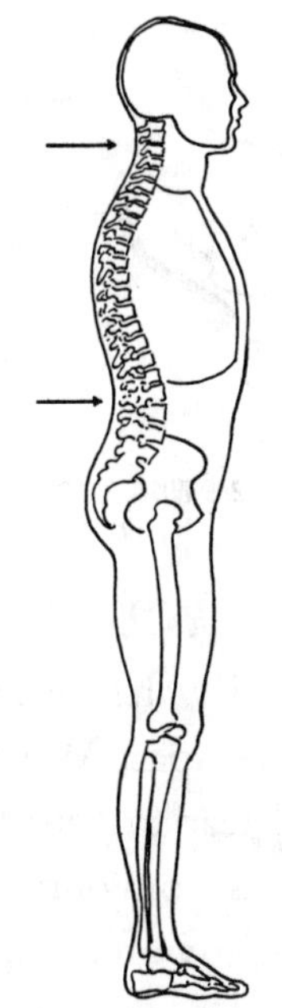

Fig. 2-7. Normal curves of the spine

Spinal nerves leave the spinal cord through openings between the vertebrae and behind the disc (Fig. 2-9). Located on the backside of these openings are the spinal joints. The extent and variety of movements of a vertebra are influenced by the shape and direction of the spinal joints. For example, the design of the spinal joints in the neck allows more forward and backward motion than in the joints of the upper mid-back vertebrae.

Muscles are the main source of force resulting in motion of the vertebrae. Six basic forms of movement are allowed within the spine: forward bending, backward bending, right and left side bending, and right and left twisting (rotation) or combinations of these.

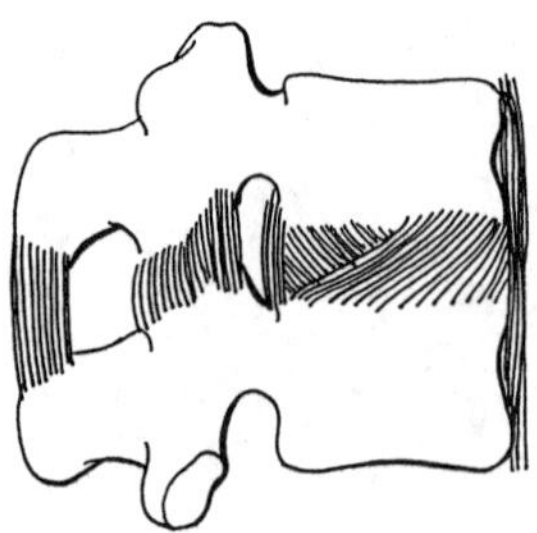

Fig. 2-8. Spinal ligaments

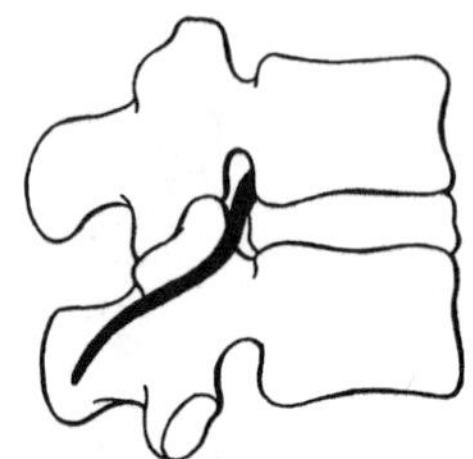

Fig. 2-9.Nerve and spinal joints

In summary, the bones, discs, and ligaments provide structure in the spine. The joints and muscles are designed for movement to occur, while every movement is coordinated by the nervous system. This coordinated effort by your nervous system regulates a balance among your muscles. Having balanced muscles throughout your body is the best protection from normal wear and tear to your spine. Balanced and strong muscles help your bones to remain strong, allow normal movement in your joints, and absorb more of the weight bearing away from the ligaments and discs in your back, helping to prevent your discs, bones, and joints from degenerating prematurely.

YOUR LIFESTYLE AND DEGENERATING BACK

By the term degenerating, I don't mean to imply that you're falling apart. What I am saying is that your daily habits can cause wear and tear to your back. Individually, we acquire certain body movements from our work and activities at home. These movements done regularly affect our muscle reflexes (nervous system) and create our muscles to develop in a certain pattern. As a result, you may have created some muscle imbalances, which, if left unchecked for long periods of time, can result in degenerative changes to your back.

How frequently does wear and tear to the spine occur? According to *The New England of Journal of Medicine*, 64 percent of adults examined with no symptoms have disc abnormalities, while eight percent of these "healthy" adults have wear and tear to their spinal joints. The older the person, the more common the degeneration. Autopsy has shown tearing of the disc in 40 percent of those between 50 and 60 years of age and in 75 percent for those between 60 and 70.

Wear and tear of the spine in itself doesn't always produce pain, yet it does make the back more susceptible to further damage. Eventually, enough damage occurs to alter the normal mechanics and function of the muscles, ligaments, discs, and joints of the back. This altered function is usually the culprit of back pain that is acquired without an injury or illness.

Altered function in the back isn't always from wear and tear. Muscle imbalances from your lifestyle can create a loss of normal function of the back. This disturbance alone can alter normal function (dysfunction) to your joints and muscles which can lead to sprains or strains, thereby causing symptoms. This is why back pain is found in both the young and the old.

For your back to function normally, you need to prevent these muscle imbalances and minimize the wear and tear to your spine. This is accomplished best by preventing the known risk factors of back pain within your lifestyle (discussed in the next chapter).

CHAPTER 3

Risk Factors for Back Pain

BACK PAIN HAS REACHED epidemic proportions within the United States. It is estimated that 208 million, or eight out of ten, Americans will experience back pain sometime in their life. In addition, it is estimated that at any given time, some 31 million Americans have low-back pain.

Fortunately, 85 percent of those suffering back pain recover within three months. However, 15 percent do not; these sufferers develop disabling back pain and become unresponsive to any form of therapy. A back disability can mean constant pain for the rest of one's life. Needless to say, this type of suffering would severely limit one's quality of life. For unknown reasons, the rate of disabling back pain is estimated to be growing at 14 times that of the total U.S. population growth. This growth rate of disability is greater than any other, including those for heart disease and arthritis.

Even those individuals who recovered from an initial severe back injury within a short time were found almost four times more predisposed to develop recurrence. It is not surprising that many researchers and health care providers are recommending that prevention of back pain must be a priority and should aim at reducing occurrence while decreasing the rate of disability.

Dealing with back dysfunction can take one of two approaches. The most common is the treatment approach, which focuses on after-injury services to help relieve and prevent recurring back pain. For example, you develop back pain, and your doctor treats the condition with a certain type of therapy (medication, manipulation, surgery, etc.) to relieve pain. In addition, your doctor, might recommend rehabilitation (back school, physical therapy, work hardening, etc.) to help prevent future occurrences.

The second approach doesn't wait for pain to develop. It is called a primary prevention approach, and it works to promote your health by positively influencing certain risk factors that may contribute to back pain or dysfunction.

Scientifically, the exact cause of all back pain is still unknown. Many people have commonly associated accidents or falls, certain diseases, and a history of back problems as causes for back pain, although researchers have found other factors associated with an increased risk of back pain. Table 3-1 categorizes these risk factors into four areas: individual, occupational, psychological, and recreational.

Research has found a person's age to have the highest correlation in developing back pain, while smoking, performing heavy work, and repetitive strain follow the lead. Risk factors for the back are similar to risk factors for heart disease in that having one or many risk factors doesn't always mean you will develop this condition. There are those who fortunately don't develop any pain, but the majority exposed to these risk factors unfortunately will. Some individuals who develop back pain may have only one risk factor, yet most people will have multiple risk factors that create more wear and tear or dysfunction to the back, eventually resulting in back pain. The key, therefore, to preventing back pain is to eliminate or minimize as many of these risk factors as possible.

TABLE 3-1
BACK-PAIN RISK FACTORS

Individual
Age
Smoking
Lack of muscle strength
Lack of flexibility
Lack of conditioning
Being overweight or tall
Improper posture
Multiple pregnancies
Changes from birth
Certain health conditions

Psychological
Pain tolerance
Anxiety
Emotional stress
Illness behavior
Job dissatisfaction

Occupational
Heavy physical work
Injury or accidents
Frequent bending, twisting, lifting, pushing or pulling
Repetitive strain
Nonmoving work postures
Vibrations

Recreational
Hockey
Rodeo riding
Football/rugby
Gymnastics
Golf
Javelin throwing
Racquetball
Bowling
Squash
Handball
Tennis
Backpacking
Rowing/kayaking
Jogging
Cross-country skiing
Wrestling
Baseball/softball

As you will learn in Chapter 5, the back-friendly workout is the only back-pain prevention tool that eliminates or minimizes each of the aforementioned risk categories of back pain. Therefore, if you don't exercise, you will be exposed to more risk, further creating more wear and tear or dysfunction to your back as you age. This book presents other back-building tips that can help you to work to minimize or eliminate the known risk factors that may contribute to back pain. Before beginning with the back-building tips, however, let's further discuss each category of risk factors so that you will become aware of the known hazards to your back.

INDIVIDUAL RISK FACTORS

Women appear to have a high risk with **advancing age** due to osteoporosis (brittle bone disease). Brittle bone disease occurs when the body's bones lose the minerals that build bones strong. When these minerals are lost, bones become weak or brittle, even to the point where the vertebrae collapse upon each other and create a hump in the back (Fig. 3-1). In women, this usually occurs years after menopause. Men are more likely to develop a herniated disc and are twice as likely as women to require surgery for this problem. The common age for this type of surgery is between 40 and 45. Obviously, as we age, more wear and tear can occur to our back, eventually causing back pain.

Smoking is a high-risk factor for developing back pain. Since smoking decreases the amount of oxygen to the discs, it increases the likelihood of disc degeneration. Also, some smokers tend to cough fre-

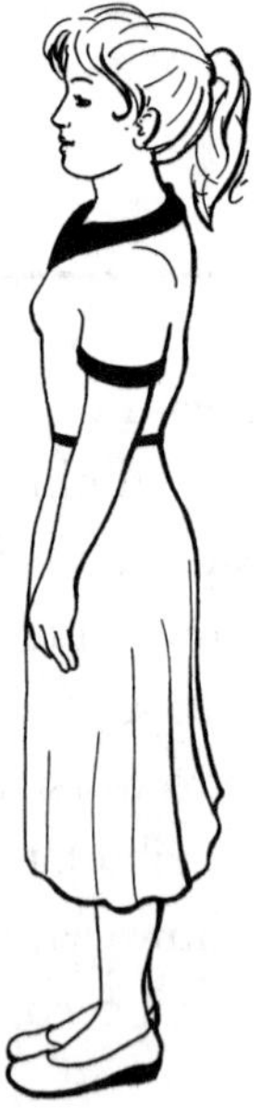

Fig. 3-1a. Young woman

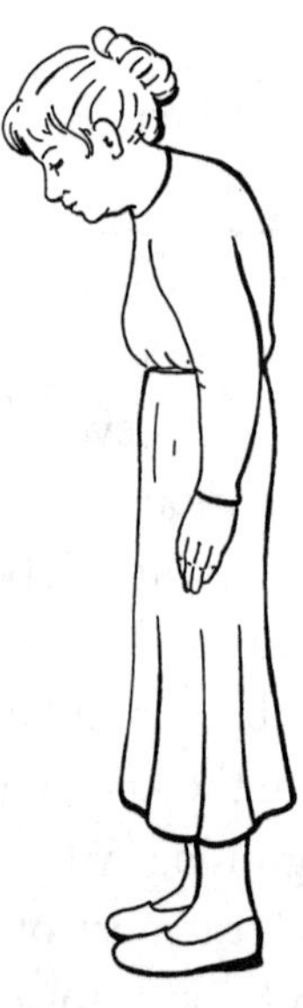

Fig. 3-1b. Elderly woman with osteoporosis

quently because of bronchitis and the dreaded "smoker's cough," causing repetitive strain upon the back.

Decreased **muscular strength** has been associated with an increased likelihood of developing low-back pain. People with back pain often have little strength in their abdominal and back muscles. Individuals with a low level of **conditioning** and **flexibility** are more likely to develop pain than those who are fit.

With regards to **body composition**, there are two individual body types of concern. Being tall or obese has been shown by some studies to increase one's risk of back pain. It is not quite known why tall people tend to have more back pain, but it can be assumed that tall people may have a harder time maintaining good posture when standing or sitting. In addition, because they are bigger, they often tend to believe they are more capable of lifting or doing manual labor, which may increase their risk. Obese individuals, especially men, tend to carry their extra weight around their midsection. Having a protruding belly changes one's center of gravity and creates abnormal weight-bearing to the spine, thus creating more dysfunction to the back. Obviously, being obese creates a heavier and constant load upon the spine, again making one more susceptible to wear and tear.

Women with **multiple pregnancies** are at risk for several reasons. First, women experience a loss of abdominal muscle tone following pregnancy. Abdominal muscles help support the back and maintain good posture. Second, women's bodies are obviously stretched during pregnancy. The ligaments of a woman's body become very flexible. As noted in the previous chapter, ligaments hold bones and joints together. It is believed that after multiple pregnancies, these ligaments become loose and allow more wear and tear within the spine. It is also believed that more wear and tear may occur to the spine during these multiple pregnancies.

As a parent, I'm well aware that having kids requires me to lift, carry, and bend more than I did before my children were born. Of course, my wife and I would never want to eliminate this interaction with our children, but we do try to minimize these improper move-

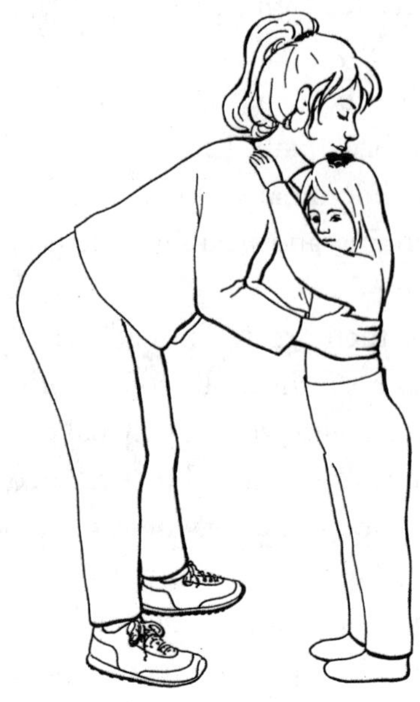

Fig. 3-2a. Incorrect lifting of children

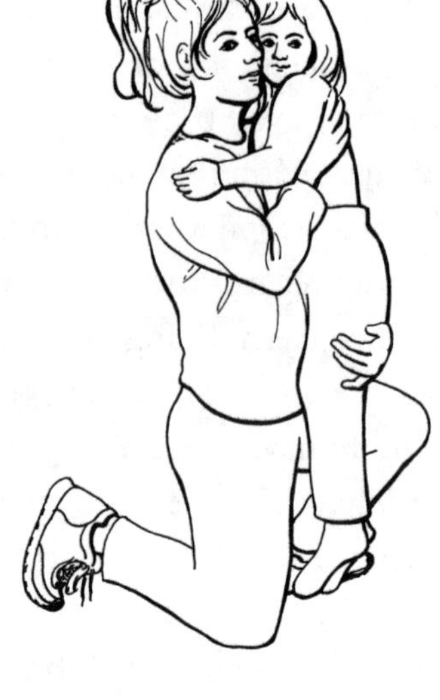

Fig. 3-2b. Correct lifting of children

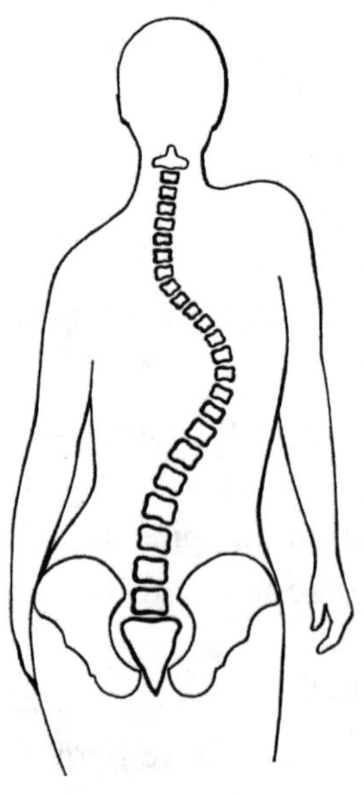

Fig. 3-3. Scoliosis

ments whenever possible (Fig. 3-2). This increased rate of lifting and carrying children obviously increases with the number of children one has and with the increased time spent with small children.

Surprisingly, general **postural deformities** are considered of minor significance as a risk factor for back pain, the exception being severe scoliosis (Fig. 3-3), which has been associated with an increased risk. An increased forward curve in the low back or a rounded hunchback curve in the mid-back has been found to appear frequently with individuals suffering from back pain. Unequal leg length doesn't seem to be a significant risk to your back, although I wouldn't advise you to start jogging if one of your legs is shorter than the other.

Some people are born with conditions that might put them at risk for back pain. Such conditions include a narrowed opening in the spine for either the spinal cord or spinal nerve roots. Other abnormal structural changes may be present in the joints, discs, and vertebrae. Certain diseases, such as infections to the spinal area, may pose a risk to back pain. In addition, certain types of cancer develop or spread to the spine that will also cause pain. Luckily, these conditions and changes from birth are relatively rare in the overall development of back pain. Table 3-2 lists some examples of **health conditions** that can cause back pain.

TABLE 3-2

HEALTH CONDITIONS THAT CAN CAUSE BACK PAIN

(INDIVIDUAL OR IN COMBINATION)

Certain Diseases	**Infections**
Scheuermann's disease	Meningitis
Paget's disease	Osteomyelitis
Kidney disease	Tuberculous spondylitis
Nutritional Diseases	**Arthritis**
Osteoporosis	Osteoarthritis
Osteomalacia	Reiter's syndrome
	Ankylosing spondylitis
Cancers Related to the Spine	**Structural changes**
Multiple myeloma	Spinal stenosis
Prostate (advanced)	Scoliosis
Breast (advanced)	Spondylolisthesis
Hodgkin's disease (advanced)	Ruptured disc
	Fusion of the vertebrae (in part or whole)

OCCUPATIONAL RISK FACTORS

Certain postures and work activities place excessive mechanical demands upon your body. These physical work factors have been found to be associated with the development of back injuries.

Jobs that require **heavy physical work** have significantly higher rates of back injuries. Occupations that require large amounts of manual handling (lifting), such as laborers, trash collectors, and nurses, are at a very high risk. Several other studies have shown that people handling heavy loads while at work experience back pain almost twice as often as those working in light occupations.

Certain body movements play a role in the increased risk of back pain. The three worst movements are twisting, repetitive bending, and reaching for or carrying objects away from the body. Pushing and pulling and arching of the low back have also been found to be problematic. These body movements should be eliminated or minimized not only at work but also at home or when participating in a recreational activity. In fact, all fitness programs have these movements incorporated into their workouts. The back-friendly workout, discussed in Chapters 7-10, will be your guide to getting a good workout with minimal, if any, improper back movements.

Repetitive strain has been shown to be detrimental to your back. Such strain can occur with frequent bending and twisting, usually associated with lifting, although lifting doesn't necessarily have to be involved. For example, repetitive strain can be associated with jobs that require asymmetric (using one side of your body) postures with no lifting.

By now you may be thinking nonphysical jobs are the best for your back. This is not necessarily so. **Nonmoving postures,** such as long-term sitting, have repeatedly been shown to lead to increased back pain. This may be because pressure within the disc during sitting is significantly higher than during standing. Think of your dentist, who throughout the day sits and leans forward to treat his or her patients' teeth. Even though your dentist isn't doing heavy work, he or she still sits, bends forward, and twists repetitively. Done over a long period of time, this is a risk to your back. Jobs that require long-term, nonmoving, standing positions (E.g., road flaggers) have also been found to put one's back at risk.

Driving a motor vehicle is even more harmful than just sitting because it involves the combination of sitting and **vibrational forces**. Commuters and other drivers who drive more than two hours a day are twice as likely to damage a disc as those who spend less time in their vehicle. Male truck drivers have been found four times more likely than other men to develop disc injuries. Vibration has an effect on the back in several ways. It can cause changes that include muscular fatigue, an increased rate of wear and tear, arthritis, loss of minerals to the bones, and decreased bloodflow to the spine. Therefore, individuals whose job (such as someone who operates a jackhammer) exposes them to vibrational forces are at risk.

Back **injuries** and **accidents** are common within the workplace and can develop from a fall or a vehicle accident or by slipping or overloading the back when lifting. Of course, injuries and accidents do occur away from work. You can be involved in an automobile accident or injure yourself at home or when participating in a recreational event.

RECREATIONAL RISK FACTORS

As mentioned under "Individual Risks," one's physical condition is associated with the development of back pain. A physically fit person is less likely to have an initial episode of back pain, and if back pain has already developed, it is less likely to recur in a physically fit person. Yet, it is important to choose the proper way to achieve physical fitness because certain sports and recreational activities can increase one's risk of developing back pain.

I'm aware that you might perceive many of the recreational activities discussed in the following section as being uncommon, done only among our youth, or not applicable to your geographical region. Since each person and each place are unique, I will list each recreational risk factor. I would hate to have anybody develop back pain because he or she was uninformed of the risk of a certain recreational activity. Remember, what is common in your area might not be common in others. For example, it is not unusual to find adult hockey players in Canada, rodeo riders in Texas, or rugby players in England. Don't forget about our youth, who may wrestle or throw the javelin for the local high school team. I encourage you to read the entire section and not read about just the activities that interest you. By being knowledgeable of all activities, you might be able to help educate others about their possible risk.

Activities To Avoid

Golf and **tennis** have been associated with an increased risk of disc injuries causing back pain as a result of the twisting movements that these sports require. As a general rule, I advise people to stay away from recreational activities that use only one side of the body, such as **racquetball, squash, handball,** and **bowling.** These sports create twisting movements that will weaken the structure of the discs. The risk of **baseball** and **softball** occurs from twisting during batting. Repetitive swinging of a bat can create back pain, most commonly in the low back. In addition, softball and baseball players tend to throw repetitively using one side of the body, putting their spine further at risk.

When I talk about **rodeo riding,** I'm not referring to people who drive their cars along Rodeo Drive in Beverly Hills. I'm talkin' 'bout the rough and tough cattle and horse riders, who truly are rough and tough. I don't know how a rider can last a year, let alone a whole career! Rodeo riders must have a high tolerance for pain, because injury is part of this sport. The danger to the back comes from the falls, bull and bronco riding, and steer wrestling.

Several athletic activities have been found to put people at risk for separation of a vertebra (**spondylolysis**) or to cause the front part of the vertebrae to displace forward (**spondylolisthesis**), putting further strain upon the spinal nerves (Fig. 3-4). These activities include **football, rugby, gymnastics, javelin throwing, backpacking, crew, rowing,** and **hockey**. Players in collision sports, such as rugby, foot-

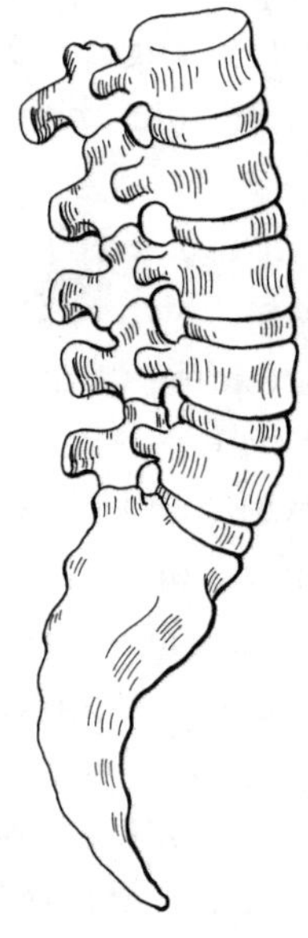

Fig. 3-4a.Normal low back spine

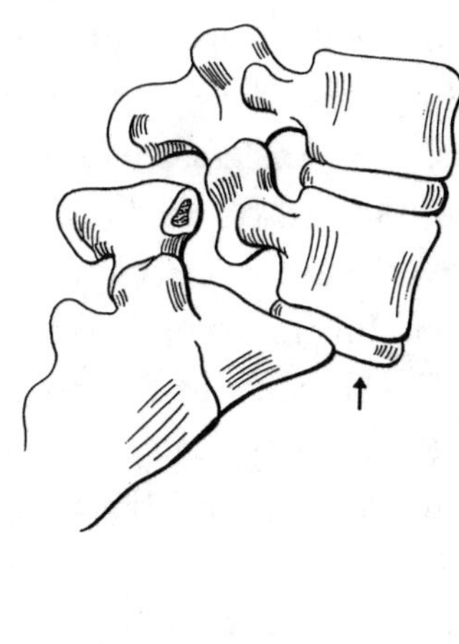

Fig. 3-4b. Spondylolisthesis

ball, and hockey, also have an increased likelihood of developing premature and advanced (wear and tear) arthritis within the spine.

Not only is hockey a rough sport with body blocks and endless falls, but it also involves two repetitive movements that harm the back. When skating, a hockey player must lean forward to gain speed. This constant forward lean puts excessive pressure upon the back, creating more wear and tear. To make matters worse, this is the same position that a player may take during a body block, creating even more damage. If that weren't bad enough, a hockey player, usually in a forward-bending position, will twist the upper body to strike the puck. This forward bending and twisting is a dangerous combination for the back, making hockey a high-risk factor for developing back pain.

The greatest risk to the spine among hockey players is to the neck. Hockey players are about three times as likely as football players to develop a severe spinal injury with paralysis. Both hockey and football athletes make contact with their head to deliver or receive a block. This could lead to a fracture in the neck and possible paralysis. Unlike hockey, organized football has made rule changes to help prevent this type of injury from occurring. These rule changes have helped to reduce severe spinal injury.

Jogging and **cross-country skiing** are controversial as being risk factors. Nevertheless, these activities have been shown to be a problem with regards to the back. The constant pounding during jogging has always been suspected as a cause of back pain. The discs absorb this pounding to the back. A healthy disc can withstand extreme compressional forces. But what about a person in his or her later years, when the discs typically aren't as strong? Or what about those with previous back injuries? If you insist on jogging, consult with your doctor first. I've seen people in their 30s with discs of a 60-year-old, and on occasion, I've seen 60-year-olds with discs of a 30-year-old. It all depends upon one's exposure to the multiple risks related to one's back.

The problem with cross-country skiing is in the arm movements. Forward arm movements away from the body are a risk. These movements also create twisting in the mid-back which is another risk. These simple movements done repetitively worry many back experts. Cross-country skiing machines aren't the only type of exercise equipment that have this forward arm movement. A number of stationary bikes have handle bars that move forward. It is best to avoid this type of equipment.

The difficulty in determining risk among recreational activities is that the environment is often uncontrolled and not easily recordable. As a result, physical and emotional stress in sports cannot always be accurately determined. Does this mean that jogging is not a risk factor for back pain? We'll have to wait and see. Although it is possible, there are other athletic activities that might contribute to the risk of back pain that haven't yet been determined. A recent study suggests that retired **wrestlers** have a higher frequency of low-back pain than ordinary people of the same age. It was also found that retired wrestlers have a higher rate of impaired back mobility.

PSYCHOLOGICAL RISK FACTORS

Some people seem to tolerate pain better than others. This **pain behavior** becomes evident when individuals injure their back. For example, two people with similar injuries may develop completely different levels of symptoms ranging from minimal to severe pain. Regardless of whether a person injures his or her back, breaks a bone, or has a needle injection to withdraw blood, each person will have a different tolerance for pain.

Work studies have shown that individuals who perceive their work to be **emotionally stressful**, demanding, **anxiety** producing, or **less satisfying** report more low-back injuries than those who do not have such perceptions. People who are under stress, have fear, and aren't satisfied while at work are less likely to concentrate on their job tasks. This lack of concentration can lead to an injury, especially during physical labor.

It has also been documented that when back disability is involved, personal, legal, and economic factors may become more important than pain factors. In such situations, it is well-known that an **illness behavior** can develop as a result of fear and anxiety combined with prolonged inactivity. In addition, with the passage of time, individuals may elaborate and exaggerate their symptoms. A good example of illness behavior occurs when a person is involved in a car accident or is hurt on the job and suffers a truly severe injury. Even after some treatment, the person's physician finds a permanent level of damage or disability to the person's back. Yet, when an injured person begins to worry and have fears of developing pain while doing certain tasks around the house or at work that he or she is capable of doing, an illness behavior has occurred. Since such people have remained inactive and haven't tested their physical limits, they have underestimated what they're capable of doing and worry unnecessarily. In addition, possibly under the advice of an attorney, a person may have been instructed to exaggerate his or her pain and limitations in order to get a larger settlement. In such a case, pain factors and perceived limitations are actually greater than the disability because of legal and economic factors.

CONCLUSION

The risks of back pain are many, although it's your exposure to these risks that increases the likelihood of developing a back condition. The next chapter provides you with a guide to determine your own personal exposure to a number of risk factors. Knowing your risk exposure is your first step to building a better back.

CHAPTER 4

Assessing Your Risk for Back and Neck Pain

MOST BACK AND NECK PAIN are the result of an accumulation of repetitive risks placed upon the spine and not from a single injury or condition. This overload of risk is usually the result of frequent exposure to a number of back-pain risk factors associated with one's daily lifestyle. Obviously, the more you're exposed to different types or combinations of risk factors, the more likely back pain will occur. Although there are no absolutes, even being exposed to one risk factor on a repetitive basis can lead to back pain.

The key to a back-pain prevention program is to assess your exposure to the risks and then find a way to eliminate or minimize such exposure. With that in mind, complete the following questionnaire. The questions are only a guideline of your possible risk exposure that could lead to wear and tear or dysfunction in your back. They are not indicative of the only way you can develop back pain. Nor is it guaranteed that exposure to these risks will create back pain. The information in the questionnaire is designed to help you to determine your exposure to certain known risks associated with back pain. Through this information you will know where to make changes to minimize your risk.

This questionnaire was developed from the scientific literature and by my professional experience. The following point system was based primarily on the literature. High risk factors or effective preventive approaches were given greater point values, while low risk factors and lesser effective preventive approaches were given lower values.

INDIVIDUAL RISK FACTORS

1. Age

35-55	56 & up	18-34
20	15	5

Points ________

2. Smoking

Cigarettes per Day

1-5	6-10	11-20	21 or more
5	10	20	30

Points ________

3. Exercise

If you already participate in the back-friendly workout, no points will be added to the next three questions. However, if you don't participate in this workout program, you'll need to add the appropriate points. If you currently stretch, weight train, or participate in a conditioning workout, finish reading this book before answering the following three questions. If you aren't doing any of the above activities, go ahead and answer questions A, B, and C.

A. Do you participate in a regular full-body weight-training workout two to three times a week?

Yes	No
5	10

Points ________

B. Do you participate in a regular full-body stretching routine four to five times a week?

Yes	No
5	10

Points ________

C. Do you participate in a regular conditioning workout at least three times a week for about 20-30 minutes?

Yes	No
5	10

Points ________

4. Do you always wear a seat belt while in a motor vehicle?

Yes	No
0	5

Points ________

5. Are you tall?

Men:

5′10″- 6′0″	over 6′0″- 6′2″
1 pt.	2 pts.
over 6′2″- 6′4″	over 6′4″
3 pts.	4 pts.

Points ________

Women:

5′5″- 5′7″	over 5′7″- 5′9″
1 pt.	2 pts.
over 5′9″- 5′11″	over 5′11″
3 pts.	4 pts.

Points ________

6. Are you overweight? Check the weight chart in Table 4-1. To determine your body frame, measure the circumference of your wrist. Then match your wrist size below to body frame in Table 4-1.

Women:

Small	Medium	Large
less than 5 1/4"	5 1/4-6"	more than 6"

Men:

Small	Medium	Large
less than 6 1/4"	6 1/4-7"	more than 7"

Overweight by

< 10 %	10-19%	20-29%	30-39 %	40 % or >
1 pt.	2 pts.	3 pts.	4 pts.	5 pts.

Points________

For example if you're a 5'7", 198-lb. man with a large body frame, you're 30 pounds overweight. You will then need to divide 30 by 168, and you'll get .1785. If you round that off, you get 18 percent. This percentage will give you two points.

TABLE 4-1

WEIGHT CHART FOR MEN AND WOMEN

Men

Height Feet	Inches	Small Frame	Medium Frame	Large Frame
5	2	128-134	131-141	138-150
5	3	130-136	133-143	140-153
5	4	132-138	135-145	142-156
5	5	134-140	137-148	144-160
5	6	136-142	139-151	146-164
5	7	138-145	142-154	149-168
5	8	140-148	145-157	152-172
5	9	142-151	148-160	155-176
5	10	144-154	151-163	158-180
5	11	146-157	154-166	161-184
6	0	149-160	157-170	164-188
6	1	152-164	160-174	168-192
6	2	155-168	164-178	172-197
6	3	158-172	167-182	176-202
6	4	162-176	171-187	181-207

Source: Metropolitan Life Insurance Company.

Women

Height Feet	Inches	Small Frame	Medium Frame	Large Frame
4	10	102-111	109-121	118-131
4	11	103-113	111-123	120-134
5	0	104-115	113-126	122-137
5	1	106-118	115-129	125-140
5	2	108-121	118-132	128-143
5	3	111-124	121-135	131-147
5	4	114-127	124-138	134-151
5	5	117-130	127-141	137-155
5	6	120-133	130-144	140-159
5	7	123-136	133-147	143-163
5	8	126-139	136-150	146-167
5	9	129-142	139-153	149-170
5	10	132-145	142-156	152-173
5	11	135-148	145-159	155-176
6	0	138-151	148-162	158-179

Source: Metropolitan Life Insurance Company.

The table lists weight in pounds for men and women, age 25 to 59, in indoor clothing. Weights are according to height, including one-inch heels, with five pounds of clothing for men and three pounds of clothing for women.

7. Determine your risk for lifting and carrying at home and during leisure (not weight-training) activities. First, approximate the maximum weight you can lift of certain objects at home. Then look at the chart in Table 4-2 to determine whether the objects are categorized at 5%, 25%, 50%, or 75% of your maximum lifting capacity. At this point, you need to determine how often during the day you lift and/or carry an object.

   If you lift and carry multiple size objects, try to determine an average in time. For example, let's say you have three children, ages 5, 3, and 18 months. In the morning and evening hours during the week and throughout the weekend, you find yourself doing a lot of lifting and carrying. Understandably, you lift and carry the 18-month-old more than the 3-year-old, and the 3-year-old more than the 5-year-old.

   On an average per day, you lift and carry the 18-month-old between one and two hours. You lift and carry both the 3-year-old and the 5-year-old less than an hour per day. You estimate your maximum lifting capacity for lifting children to be 100 pounds. Since your 18-month-old weighs 26 pounds, your 3-year-old 35 pounds, and your 5-year-old 52 pounds, you can determine what category each child will be listed under. The 18-month-old is considered an occasional moderate lift on the chart in Table 4-2, for a total of 2 points; the 3-year-old is considered a moderate lift, giving you an additional 2 points, while your 5-year-old is considered a heavy lift, for 3 points.

In addition to taking care of your children, you cook and clean the house about an hour a day on an average. During these activities, you lift and carry at approximately 5% to 10% of your maximum lifting capacity. Therefore, you'll need to add another point to your total for lifting and carrying points, giving you a total of 8 points.

TABLE 4-2

RISK FOR LIFTING AND CARRYING AT HOME

	TIME				
	1 hour or less	Occasional 1-2 hours	Intermittent 2-4 hours	Frequent 4-6 hours	Constant 6-8 hours
5-10% Minimal	1	1.5	2	3	3.5
11-25% Light	1.5	2	2-3	3-4	4-5
26-50% Moderate	2	2-3	4-5	4-6	5-7
51-75% Heavy	3	3-4	4-6	7-10	10-15
76% & up Very Heavy	3.5	4-5	5-7	10-15	20-30
Points					

Total Points ________

8. Determine your risk for movements during nonwork activities (except for athletic activities listed under recreational risk factors). You need to analyze your movements while off work to determine which you do frequently. You may have one movement or multiple movements to correlate to a time frame.

   If needed, copy the list of activities in Table 4-3 and keep it with you. If your activities vary from day to day, it may be helpful for you to add your total hours of specific movements for the week and then divide by 7 to get a daily average. For example, Mike is a mail carrier and former mechanic. To earn extra money, he begins to work on cars in his garage during the evening and on weekends. Mike quickly becomes busy with his side work, averaging three hours a day working on engines. Mike has exposed himself to a number of repetitive improper movements. For starters, he bends forward for approximately two hours (3 points), reaches outward (2 points) for about an hour a day, and twists (3 points) for about an hour a day.

In addition, Mike is an avid sports fan. Whether it is football, basketball, or baseball season, Mike can be found sitting in front of the TV in his favorite chair. Between viewing sports and watching his favorite shows, he spends about 18 hours a week watching TV, giving him an average of about two and a half hours a day (2.5 points). Mike's home and leisure activities thus give him a risk total of 10.5 points.

TABLE 4-3

MOVEMENTS DURING NONWORK ACTIVITIES

(Cross off the appropriate point box)

Activity	Number of hours per day 1 hr.	2 hrs.	3 hrs.	4 hrs.	5 hrs.	6 hrs.	7 hrs.	8 hrs.
Twisting	3	4	5	6	7	8	9	10
Bending forward	2	3	4	5	6	7	8	9
Reaching outward	2	3	4	5	6	7	8	9
Bending backward	1	2	3	4	5	6	7	8
Sitting	1	2	3	4	5	6	7	8
Driving	1	2	3	4	5	6	7	8
One-sided movements	1	2	3	4	5	6	7	8
Pushing & pulling	0	0	1	2	3	4	5	6
Standing	0	0	0	0	0	1	2	3
Average Daily Points								

* Driving includes, noncommute driving of cars, trucks, or recreational vehicles.

Total Points ________

DETERMINING ADDITIONAL RISK FOR WOMEN

Osteoporosis is one of most common and feared conditions of the elderly. This condition mainly affects women, since women have 30 percent less peak bone mass than men and experience hormonal changes following menopause, although some women are at greater risk than others.

Osteoporosis is a condition wherein bones become brittle. These brittle bones can create fractures, most commonly in the hips, spine, and wrists. In the spine, the bones can become so weak that they are unable to hold one's body weight and may collapse as the result of a simple activity such as sneezing, or stepping off a curb. This collapse occurs most commonly in the mid-back region. The main cause of osteoporosis in women is the lack of the hormone estrogen after menopause, which leads to a rapid loss of calcium in the bones for five to ten years. Calcium helps to make the bones strong and is commonly found in dairy products such as milk, yogurt, cheese and leafy green vegetables.

Because of other contributing factors, some women are at greater risk than others. The following questions will help you to determine whether you are at an increased risk for developing this condition. Smoking, age, and a lack of exercise are contributing factors. Since we already included these factors in your back-pain risk profile, you won't find them in the following questionnaire.

1. Osteoporosis risk factors

   Add one point for each yes answer. Then total your points at the end of this list. Keep in mind that you can develop osteoporosis and not have back pain. Back pain associated with osteoporosis occurs when a fracture develops in your vertebrae. Such fractures usually occur late in life. In addition, risks associated with certain diseases, immobility, age, lack of hormones, or medications have been omitted. Only the following osteoporosis risk considerations will be rated in determining your risk in the development of back pain.

A. Are you a Causcasian woman?

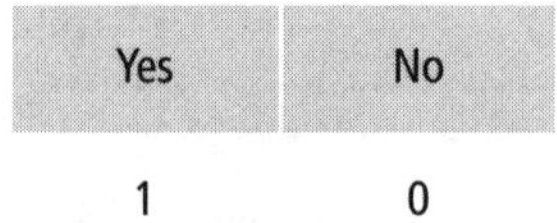

1 0

B. As a child and a young adult, did (do) you have a diet low in dairy products (milk, cheese, etc.)?

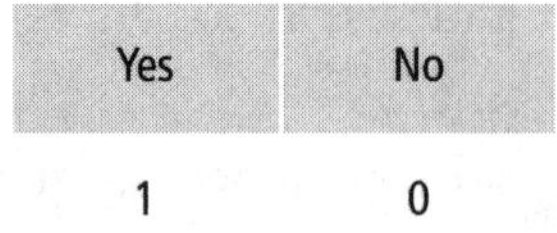

1 0

C. Do you consume a high-protein diet? Food consists of carbohydrates, protein, and fats. If you consume above 15% of your total food intake from protein, the answer is yes. Protein is found in meats, fish, beans, nuts, and dairy products.

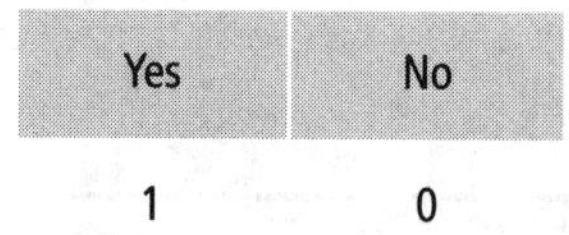

Yes	No
1	0

D. Do you consume large amounts of caffeine (more than 4 cups of coffee, tea or cola beverages per day)?

Yes	No
1	0

Total Osteoporosis Points ________

2. Multiple pregnancies:

Number of Pregnancies

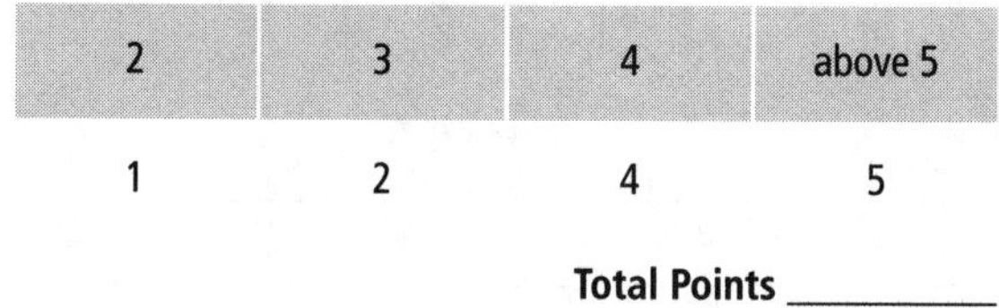

2	3	4	above 5
1	2	4	5

Total Points ________

Your total individual risk: points ________

OCCUPATIONAL RISK FACTORS

1. When determining your lifting and carrying during a typical workday, first approximate the maximum weight you can lift of certain objects at work. Then look at the chart in Table 4-4 to determine whether the objects are categorized at 5%, 25%, 50%, or 75% of your maximum lifting capacity. At this point, you need to determine how often during the day you lift and/or carry an object. If you lift and carry multiple size objects, try to determine an average in time.

For example, Norma is a nurse who works at a nursing home for the elderly. She lifts and carries people throughout the day. Norma can lift a 120-lb. person with the help of the patient or a fellow nurse; she can carry up to 80 pounds. On a typical workday, Norma estimates that she lifts or carries five hours a day. Two hours a day are spent lifting at a moderate level (3 points), one hour a day is spent lifting and carrying at a light level (1.5 points), another hour is spent lifting and

TABLE 4-4

RISK FOR LIFTING AND CARRYING AT WORK

	TIME				
	1 hour or less	Occasional 1-2 hours	Intermittent 2-4 hours	Frequent 4-6 hours	Constant 6-8 hours
5-10% Minimal	1	1.5	2	3	3.5
11-25% Light	1.5	2	2-3	3-4	4-5
26-50% Moderate	2	2-3	4-5	4-6	5-7
51-75% Heavy	3	3-4	4-6	7-10	10-15
76% & up Very Heavy	3.5	4-5	5-7	10-15	20-30
Points					

Total Points ________

carrying at a minimal level (1 point), half an hour is spent lifting at a heavy level (1.5 points), and half an hour is spent lifting at a very heavy level (1.75 points). Norma has a total risk of 8.75 points.

2. To determine whether your movements at work are at risk, you need to analyze them while at work to determine which movements you do frequently. You may have one or multiple movements to correlate to a time frame.

If needed, copy the list of movements in Table 4-5 and take it to work to help you correlate your movements to a certain time frame. For example, Curly is a carpenter who exposes himself on a daily basis to multiple improper movements. Curly specializes in building wooden frames for homes. As a result, he spends five hours a day bending forward to hammer and saw wood (6 points). Curly hammers with his right hand an average of five hours a day. This one-sided movement is a risk to Curly's neck region (5 points). When grabbing building materials and using his hammer and saw, Curly estimates that he reaches outward seven out of eight hours a day (8 points). He is also exposed to vibrational forces when using the electric saw, which he estimates that he uses about an hour and a half a day (1.5 points). Finally, Curly commutes to work a total of an hour a day (1 point). Curly's risk at work adds up to a whopping 21.5 points.

TABLE 4-5

MOVEMENTS AT WORK

(Cross off the appropriate point box)

	Number of hours per day							
Activity	**1 hr.**	**2 hrs.**	**3 hrs.**	**4 hrs.**	**5 hrs.**	**6 hrs.**	**7 hrs.**	**8 hrs.**
Twisting	3	4	5	6	7	8	9	10
Bending forward	2	3	4	5	6	7	8	9
Reaching outward	2	3	4	5	6	7	8	9
Bending backward	1	2	3	4	5	6	7	8
Sitting	1	2	3	4	5	6	7	8
Driving*	1	2	3	4	5	6	7	8
Vibrational forces (e.g. jackhammer)	1	2	3	4	5	6	7	8
One-sided movements	1	2	3	4	5	6	7	8
Pushing & pulling	0	0	1	2	3	4	5	6
Standing	0	0	0	0	0	1	2	3
Average Daily Points								

* Driving includes, cars, trucks, forklifts, or other moving equipment, both at work and commuting.

Total Points ________

Your total occupation risk: Points ________

RECREATIONAL RISK FACTORS

The more you participate in any of the activities listed in Table 4-6, the more risk you apply to your back. First, determine whether you participate in any of the following activities on a minimal (one to three times a month), an occasional (once or twice a week), or a regular (three to seven times a week) basis. Then check the appropriate box associated with your activity. For example, you may backpack on a minimal level during the summer months, golf occasionally throughout the year, and play regularly in a softball league and a hockey league.

Your next step is to figure out your annual amount of these activities. As a backpacker, you hiked twice each month during the months of June, July, and August. You would therefore mark "3" under the Annual Amount column for the minimal category, since you backpacked three separate months within the minimal category (twice a month). If you golfed for 15 weeks on an occasional basis, you would mark "15" under Annual Amount for the occasional category. Participating in league play requires that you play an average of three to four times a week, including league games, tournaments, and practices. Softball and hockey season both last 12 weeks. Therefore, you would mark "12" under Annual Amount for the regular category for softball and hockey.

Next you will multiply your frequency numbers times the minimal, occasional, and regular ratings (.1, .2, .4, .5, .6, or .8). For example, since you backpacked three separate months at a minimal level, multiply 3 times .1 for a total of .3. Continuing with the above, 15 multiplied by .5 gives you a total of 7.5, 12 multiplied by .5 gives you a total of 6, and 12 multiplied by .8 gives you a total of 9.6. The total is your annual risk, or 23.4 points.

TABLE 4-6
RECREATIONAL ACTIVITIES

	Frequency				
	Minimal	Occasional	Regular		
Activity	1-3 month	1-2 a week	3-7 a week	Annual Amount	
HOCKEY	.2	.6	.8	X	=
RODEO RIDING	.2	.6	.8	X	=
FOOTBALL/ RUGBY	.2	.6	.8	X	=
GOLF	.1	.5	.6	X	=
GYMNASTICS	.1	.5	.6	X	=
BACKPACKING	.1	.4	.5	X	=
JAVELIN THROWING	.1	.4	.5	X	=
RACQUETBALL	.1	.4	.5	X	=
BOWLING	.1	.4	.5	X	=
SQUASH	.1	.4	.5	X	=
HANDBALL	.1	.4	.5	X	=
ROWING	.1	.4	.5	X	=
JOGGING	.1	.4	.5	X	=
CROSS-COUNTRY SKIING	.1	.4	.5	X	=
WRESTLING	.1	.4	.5	X	=
BASEBALL/SOFTBALL	.1	.4	.5	X	=
TENNIS	.1	.4	.5	X	=

Your total recreational risk: Points __________

PSYCHOLOGICAL RISK FACTORS

The following questions deal with how your behavior may play a role in the development of back pain:

1. How would you describe your ability to tolerate pain?

Points

Normal	Above normal	Below normal
0 pts	-3 pts	+3 pts

Points ________

2. Do you have a high level of emotional stress at home or at work?

Yes	No
+3 pts	0 pts

Points ________

3. Do you experience anxiety frequently at work or while at home?

Yes	No
+3 pts	0 pts

Your total psychological risk: Points ________

Use the following chart to total your points in each risk category.

Your Total Points	
Individual risk total	
Occupational risk total	
Recreational risk total	
Psychological risk total	
Total Points	

Guidelines for Back Pain

Some risk	Moderate risk	High risk
< 50 pts.	50-100 pts.	> 100 pts.

NOBODY'S PERFECT

It is impossible to eliminate all risk to your back. There will always be occasions when you use your back incorrectly. Also, you can't predict whether you are going to develop certain health conditions, such as structural changes from birth, infections, traumatic fractures, or certain types of cancer related to back pain.

Your lifestyle plays a major role in the development of back pain. As with preventing heart disease, prevention of back pain consists of avoiding as many health risks as possible. The more you eliminate such risks, the less likely you will develop back pain. In addition, some of these lifestyle changes will help promote your overall health.

In the next chapter, you will learn the different preventive tools for avoiding the development of back pain. Don't wait for back pain to occur; start now to build a better back. Use these tools to begin living a healthy lifestyle and to minimize repetitive risks to your back.

CHAPTER 5

Back Building

ACCORDING TO PARENTS AND FRIENDS, preventing back pain is simple. Just bend your knees, keep your back straight, and hold objects close to your body when lifting. As you now know, incorrect lifting isn't the only risk to your back. You need to do much more than take this simple approach. Fortunately, there are many preventive tools you can use when back building, although, as you will learn in this chapter, some of these tools are more effective than others.

TOOLS FOR BUILDING A BETTER BACK

Of all the primary prevention measures for back pain, exercise is the most comprehensive, although there are other preventive measures that you can take to help eliminate or minimize the risk factors for back pain. Table 5-1 lists some tools you can use that can help to prevent back pain.

TABLE 5-1

TOOLS FOR PREVENTING BACK PAIN

1. When lifting, use your legs, maintain a straight back, and keep your arms close to your body (Fig. 5-1). When possible, have others help, or use lifting devices. Wear a lifting belt when lifting heavy objects.

2. Mother was right! It is best to stand and sit tall. Use low-back cushions while sitting. Also, try to keep your knees higher than your hips when sitting, and don't cross your legs (Fig. 5-2). Avoid or minimize prolonged standing or sitting and change positions regularly or stretch. When standing, shift your weight from one leg to the other and bend one knee so that one leg is higher than the other.
3. Avoid nicotine in all its forms, if you smoke or chew, get serious about quitting.
4. Attend a back school.
5. Lower your mental stress by attending a class or by reading a book on stress management.
6. When driving, move your car seat forward so that your knees are bent. To reduce spinal trauma from a vehicle accident, never drive without a seat belt. If possible, purchase a car with air bags, which reduce the impact of a collision.
7. Make sure to lessen the vibrational effect of your car or truck by having good shocks and tires, low-back cushions, and well-cushioned seats. Also, drive on smooth or well-paved roads.
8. Evaluate your workstation. Adjust table height and chair to a comfortable level or make other mechanical changes within your workplace. If possible, rotate job tasks with others to reduce abnormal repetitive movements.
9. Sleep on a firm mattress. Since one third of your day is spent sleeping, it makes sense to find a box spring and mattress that will give your back proper support (see Appendix A). While sleeping, it is best to lie on your side with your knees bent and a pillow between your legs (Fig. 5-3) or on your back using a support (such as a pillow) under your knees (Fig. 5-4). Do not sleep on your stomach or lie on your back with your knees straight.

Keep in mind that the more you work to incorporate these prevention tools into your lifestyle, the better your odds are at preventing back pain. Don't be afraid to seek professional help if needed, especially if you're having trouble reducing your stress level or trying to quit smoking. If you feel you're having trouble with your work environment, try finding an ergonomic specialist to evaluate your workstation. These specialists perform mechanical evaluations to help minimize a person's physical stresses while at work as well as at home. In

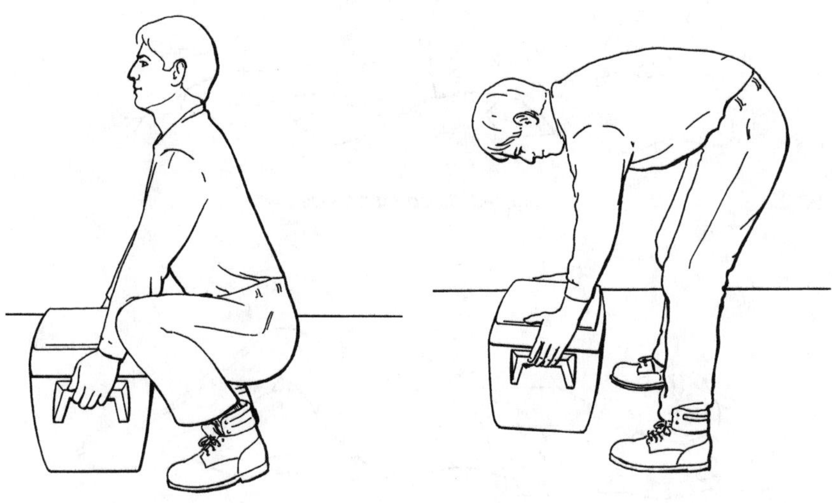

Fig. 5-1a. Correct lifting

Fig. 5-1b. Incorrect lifting

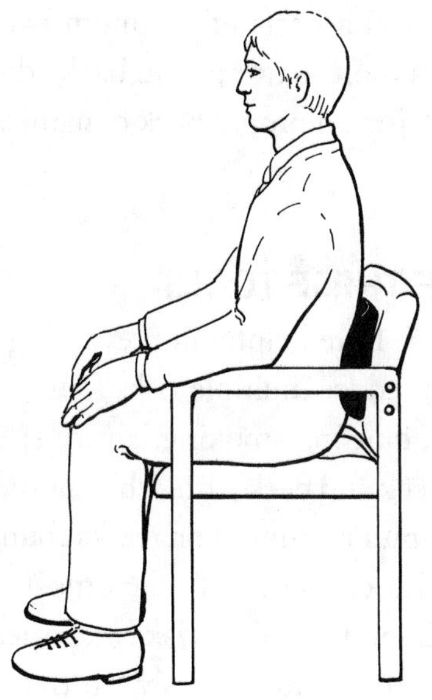

Fig. 5-2. Correct sitting

fact, one study examined the three most commonly used methods for controlling workplace back injuries (selecting the correct worker for the specific job, safe lifting training, and ergonomics) and concluded that of the three methods, only ergonomics held promise. In most instances, an ergonomic specialist is a mechanical engineer trained in this field, although many health care providers and safety personnel also have training in ergonomics.

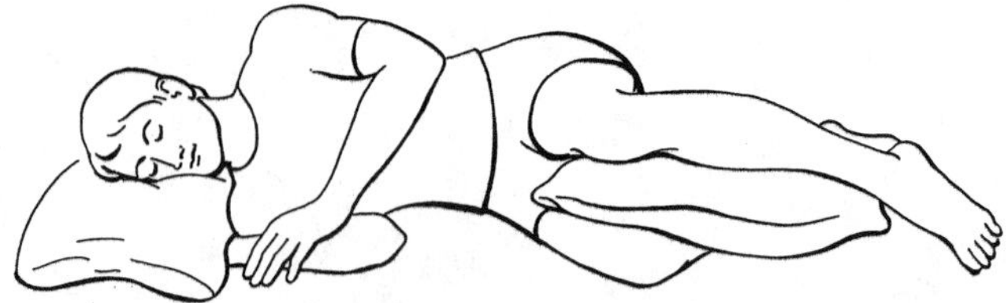

Fig. 5-3. Sleeping on side

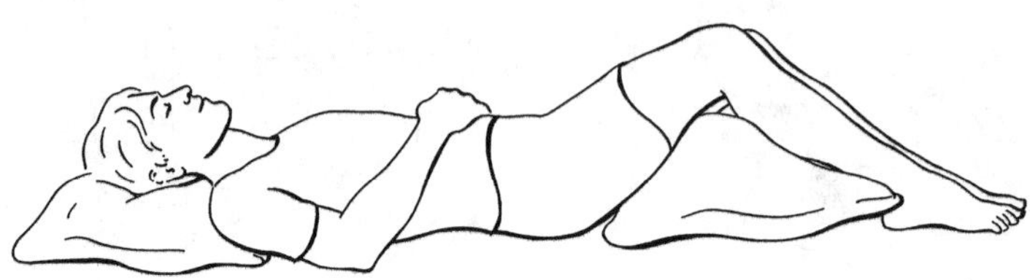

Fig. 5-4. Sleeping on back

Many hospitals and clinics offer a back school. The instructors at back schools recognize that preventive measures and an individual's responsibility for self care are two critical aspects of optimum back function. Back school programs stress a more active role in back education and conditioning, with an emphasis on proper back dynamics, body mechanics, posture, and exercise.

HOW EFFECTIVE ARE THESE TOOLS

Some of the tools listed in Table 5-1 are helpful in preventing a specific risk, while others may work to reduce multiple risks found in different risk categories. For example, quitting smoking is very specific for eliminating this high risk for neck and back pain, while proper sitting and standing techniques are helpful in minimizing risks found in both individual and occupational risk categories. In fact, most of these address risks in the occupational and individual risk categories.

Attending a back school is a bit more comprehensive in that it can minimize a number of risks found in multiple categories. Back schools usually teach the majority of the individual and occupational risks. In addition, it provides personalized instruction in and evaluation of how to lift, sit, walk, and perform a number of your daily activities. Since this instruction is usually performed by a health care provider who will critique your daily activities, it is a highly practical and recommended approach to minimizing risks.

You might also gain some psychological benefits from attending a back school. After being treated for a back injury, a person might benefit from being evaluated on the proper movements of his or her daily activities. As a result of the back injury, and prior to treatment, many of these movements may have created increased pain. Consequently, many people with back injuries are afraid to perform some of these movements because they fear it will still be painful to do so. Back schools can help to eliminate anxiety among those who have been injured and give people confidence in their ability to perform certain tasks correctly and pain free.

Unfortunately, back schools do have some drawbacks. Most back schools are designed for the individual who has injured his or her spine and not for the healthy person who wishes to prevent a back injury. Having attended many back schools, I can honestly say some are good, some not as good, and some are boring. Since there isn't any standardized instruction, I suggest you try to find a school that will at least evaluate you during some of your daily activities (lifting, mopping, shoveling, etc.). A good back school also is usually expensive and is covered by insurance only if you are recovering from a back injury and have a referral from your doctor. Finally, the exercises recommended in back schools are insufficient. These exercises usually comprise stretching and strengthening tips related to your back and posture. The healthy person needs to work out his or her entire body and not just certain parts. Therefore, a complete fitness program is needed that is designed not only for your overall health but also with regards to the risks associated with your back.

THE BEST PREVENTION TOOL

Let's see why the back-friendly workout is the single most comprehensive way to prevent back pain. As you know, the risk factors for back pain are categorized according to individual, occupational, recreational, and psychological factors. The information in Table 5-2 demonstrates how the back-friendly workout will affect all categories of the known risk factors.

As you can see the back-friendly workout can have an effect on 31 of the 37 risk factors for back pain. The following information describes how this is accomplished.

Individual Risk Factors

Your age appears to have the highest correlation in developing back pain over any other individual risk factor, although age itself might not be as great a risk as the aging process of your body. Research shows that being unfit and participating in activities that cause more wear and tear to your body will increase your susceptibility to many conditions commonly associated with aging, including developing a bad back.

Participating regularly in an exercise program not only increases your longevity but also tends to slow the aging process. Exercise helps prevent heart disease, certain types of diabetes, osteoporosis, and back strains/sprains. Also, having flexible and strong muscles, ligaments, and joints as a result of working out can help prevent back pain. By being well conditioned, you'll have a better chance of maintaining a trim physique, having well-lubricated joints and stronger bones, and having more endurance in your muscles, all of which are more conducive to maintaining a healthy back for a longer period of time.

Eliminating smoking is one of the most important preventive measures you can take to maintain your general health. Lung and other related cancers have a higher frequency rate among smokers. It is also known that smoking tends to decrease the amount of oxygen in your blood and therefore to your back. It is believed that exercise may help counteract this decrease in oxygen among smokers. Exercise may be helpful in preventing disc degeneration commonly found among those who smoke.

TABLE 5-2

EFFECTS OF THE BACK-FRIENDLY WORKOUT ON BACK PAIN RISK FACTORS

Risk Factors	Effects
Individual	Individual
1. Age	1. Slows the aging process.
2. Smoking	2. Increases the amount of oxygen and blood flow to your discs and joints of the spine.
3. Lack of muscle strength	3. Improves strength throughout your body.
4. Lack of conditioning	4. Improves your conditioning.
5. Being overweight or tall	5. Helps to maintain your proper weight.
6. Improper posture	6. Improves muscular endurance and balance needed to maintain good posture.
7. Multiple pregnancies	
8. Changes from birth	
9. Certain health conditions	
Occupational	Occupational
1. Heavy physical work	1. A fit body will help to prevent strain/sprain injuries from heavy or repetitive work, lifting, and pushing or pulling.
2. Nonmoving work postures	2. The back-friendly stretching exercises should be used at work for people with nonmoving work postures.
3. Frequent bending, twisting lifting, pushing, or pulling	3. Learning how to eliminate twisting, forward bending, and reaching from your workout may help you to avoid these movements while at work.
4. Repetitive strain	
5. Injury or accidents	
6. Vibration	
Recreational	
1. Hockey	
2. Rodeo riding	
3. Football/rugby	
4. Gymnastics	
5. Golf	
6. Javelin throwing	
7. Racquetball	
8. Bowling	
9. Squash	
10. Handball	

Recreational (cont.)

11. Tennis
12. Backpacking
13. Rowing
14. Jogging
15. Cross-country skiing
16. Wrestling
17. Baseball/softball

Psychological

1. Pain tolerance
2. Anxiety
3. Emotional stress
4. Illness behavior
5. Job dissatisfaction

Recreational

The back-friendly workout uses recreational activities that have a conditioning effect upon your body while placing minimal risk to your spine.

Psychological

1. Increases pain tolerance.
2. Helps to lower anxiety.
3. Helps to lower emotional stress.
4. Helps you to develop a healthy behavior.
5. Builds self-esteem and may improve your concentration while working.

Occupational and Recreational Risk Factors

By increasing your muscular strength, endurance, flexibility, and balance, you will be better prepared to prevent strain/sprain injuries during physical work. Weight training is essential for people whose jobs are physically demanding. Stronger muscles will absorb the heavy loads upon your back and help to reduce your risk. Your workouts will also help to counteract osteoporosis and imbalanced muscles that can develop from both work and your hobbies.

The back-friendly workout will educate you about what body movements you should avoid. By minimizing twisting and forward and backward bending, you can help prevent repetitive strain injuries both at work and when participating in recreational activities. In addition, always carry objects close to your body.

For those of you who have a nonmoving (prolonged sitting or standing) working posture, your participation in the back-friendly workout will help to counteract risk to your back. In addition, try taking a stretching break periodically while at work. This will help even more to reduce your risk for developing back pain. During work, take a moment about every hour to stretch your spine. If possible, do just one of the six cool-down exercises (discussed in Chapter 7). Then simply do a different stretch every hour.

If you are a professional or regularly participate in one of the risky recreational activities such as golf, hockey, football, or rodeo riding, it is imperative that you participate in the back-friendly workout. Working out will help minimize injuries when they occur by maintaining strength and flexibility and creating some muscle balance in your body. In other words, working out will help to counteract the stresses and strains of your particular sport. You'll also need to use the other back-building tips to reduce repetitive wear and tear to your spine and to prolong your career in these sports.

Psychological Risk Factors

Pain behavior is affected by the amount of circulating endorphins within your body. Endorphins are morphinelike hormones that are released in a variety of situations. This substance can control pain and even produce a natural feeling of well-being. It can also provide you with a sense of increased energy.

It has been shown that exercise can influence the production of endorphins within the body. It also appears that the more one exercises, the more tolerant a person becomes in accepting pain. Not surprisingly, patients with chronic (long-lasting) back pain have a low level of endorphins. When these people become active, they develop a more tolerant pain behavior, which suggests that increasing a person's activity level may play a positive role with individuals who suffer from chronic back pain.

Mental stress and anxiety are also back pain risk factors that appear to be reduced by exercise. The International Society of Sports Psychology states that conditioning exercise has been associated with reduced anxiety and stress. It appears that this reduced anxiety and stress can even carry over into the work environment, where these mental conditions have been correlated with an increased rate of back injuries. Exercise will also help you to build your self-esteem, which

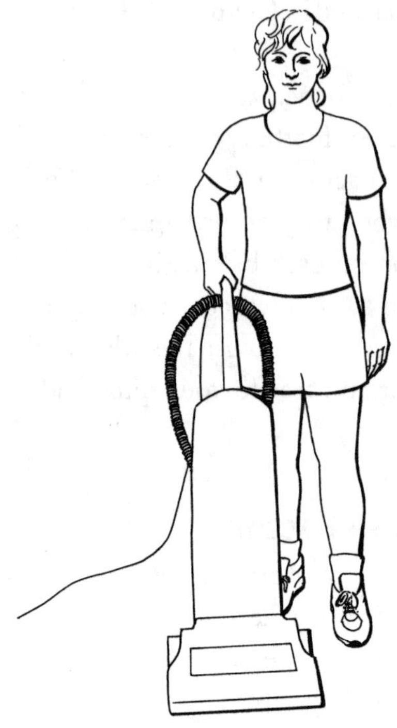

Fig. 5-5a. Correct vacuuming

will allow you to feel good about yourself. In contrast, back pain can negatively affect your employment, income, family, and social roles, producing a lack of self-esteem. By building your self-esteem and lowering your anxiety and stress, exercise may help you to feel more confident and more satisfied with your life and your work. In addition, the preceding changes may increase your concentration while you are working, thereby reducing your risk for injury.

Once an injury has occurred, prolonged inactivity has been associated with developing an illness behavior that may increase the severity of a back disability. If more people were encouraged to exercise (if permissible) after an injury, they might be able to decrease the effects of their disability. Several work studies have emphasized the need to keep people active after an injury. Allowing for a modified early return to work when capable has been shown to disrupt a person's illness behavior and allow for a faster recovery. This is significant when you consider that the increase in back disability is greater than any other type of disability, including heart disease and arthritis. In addition, back disabilities account for approximately 85 percent of the cost of back pain to our society.

As this chapter has shown, by simply participating in the back-friendly workout, you can eliminate or reduce many risks associated with back pain, although you need to make a conscious effort to avoid certain risks in your workout, such as twisting and excessive forward

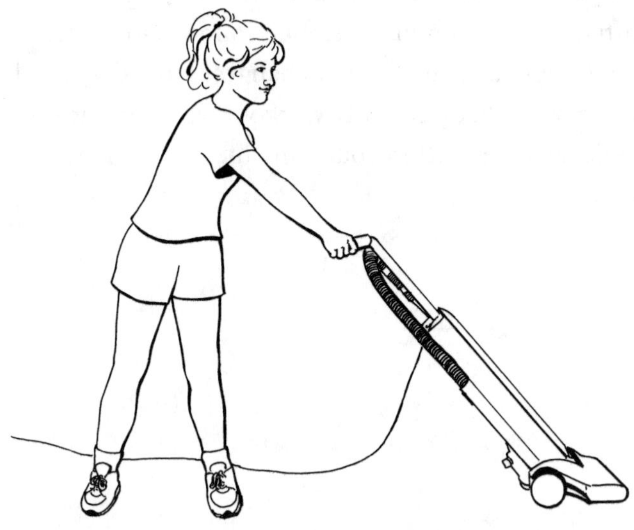

Fig. 5-5b. Incorrect vacuuming

and backward bending. To perform this workout correctly, you have no choice but to develop a healthy behavior toward the correct movements of your back. You will find that this behavior will carry over into other daily activities by helping you to be conscious of the proper movements of your back (Fig. 5-5).

TOOLS OF THE TRADE

As with all good builders, your tools are your greatest asset. The more tools you have, the better the builder you become. In addition, you always want to use the best tool for the job. As a back builder, you now know what tool is your best and how important other tools will become in building a better back.

Back pain is usually created by many factors. It is best to cover all bases by eliminating as many individual, occupational, recreational, and psychological risk factors as possible. It also appears that many of these risk factors are negotiable and can be prevented if you're willing to change your lifestyle.

Being an apprentice back builder or changing your lifestyle may sound difficult, if not impossible. The following chapter shows you how easily others have made such changes. Now that you know the broad effects of the back-friendly workout, you can learn from others how to make changes within your daily lifestyle.

CHAPTER 6

Putting It All Together

LET'S LOOK AT HOW these risk factors can apply to a person's daily lifestyle. We can show you by example how you can work to reduce or eliminate your own personal risk factors for back pain. Let's follow two fictitious examples, Connie and Otis.

CONNIE THE CAFETERIA WORKER

Connie has worked at I.M. Hurt Elementary School for the past 24 years. She is 5'9", 150 pounds, 47 years old, and married with four children.

Her job requires heavy work with repetitive bending, twisting, lifting, pushing, and pulling. A normal day begins at 6:30 a.m., when Connie is at work to receive deliveries. The driver drops all deliveries onto the kitchen floor. It's Connie's job to stack and rotate each delivery according to whether it is dry goods, produce, milk, or frozen foods. The current inventory must be rotated from the back of the refrigerator, freezer, storage room, or shelf to the front, while the new inventory is stacked behind to make sure only properly dated food is

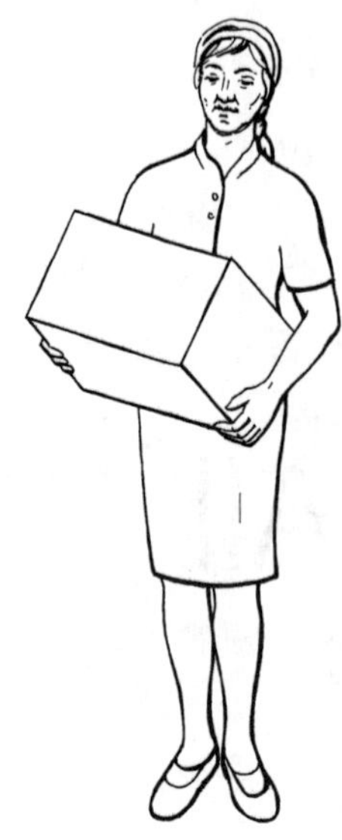

Fig. 6-1. Carrying boxes of food

used. Connie must carry 50-lb. boxes of flour and sugar to the storage room and cases of food to the freezer, both located in another building (Fig. 6-1).

After stacking inventory, Connie begins to prepare breakfast for 200 students. Today Connie and her co-workers will cook pancakes, warm up rolls, and have cereal, milk, and juice available. At 7:30, Connie begins to serve breakfast, and by 8:00 she cleans the tables while others wash the dishes. The 14 tables used by the students are short and have benches in front of them. As a result, Connie leans her tall and large-frame body forward over the bench to clean the tables by hand. Cleaning the tables also requires her to reach outward and to twist her upper body (Fig. 6-2).

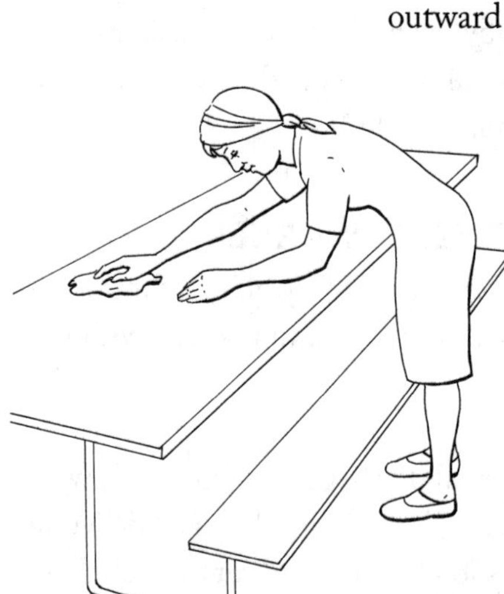

Fig. 6-2. Cleaning table incorrectly

When preparing and cooking the school lunch, Connie must lift heavy pots and trays filled with food. The trays are placed into the oven to cook the food and then are placed into the warmer until serving time. Since the ovens and warmers are multiple layered, Connie must bend and twist to push the trays of food into the lower oven or warmer (Fig. 6-3). To place food in the upper ovens or warmer, Connie must lift the trays above her head and reach outward.

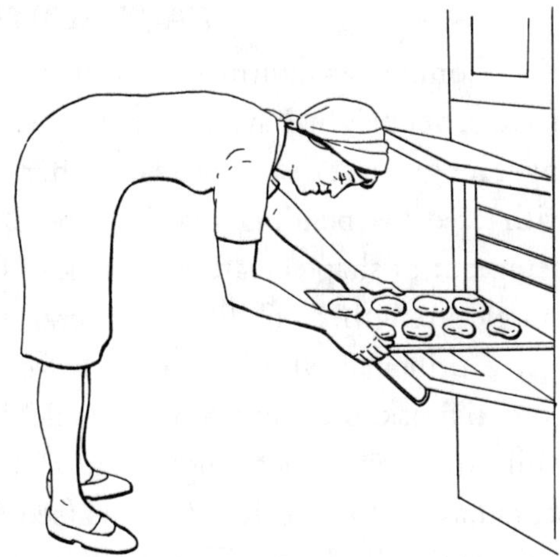

Fig. 6-3. Putting food in oven incorrectly

When lunchtime arrives, Connie must empty the heavy pots and trays into the food containers and carry them to the serving line. During serving time, her job is busy and stressful. It is the vice principal's job to monitor the children's behavior while they are waiting in line for lunch. The vice principal doesn't like to see the serving line slow down or stop because the children are more apt to misbehave. Therefore, the vice principal is constantly yelling at the kitchen staff to keep busy. Meanwhile, Connie is running back and forth from the kitchen to the serving area carrying containers of food and milk.

I.M. Hurt Elementary School feeds lunch to 400 children during two different servings. The first lunch is at 11:15, and the second at 12:15. Typically, it takes 40 minutes to serve and feed the children before Connie can begin to clean the tables and prepare for the second lunch. As a result of this time schedule, Connie must clean the tables three times a day, with only 10 minutes to clean 14 tables after the first lunch.

Finally, Connie helps with the dishes, sweeps and mops the kitchen (more twisting), and prepares food for the following day's meal. Once at home, she cooks and cleans for her family. She also goes bowling every Wednesday night with her friends.

BACK BUILDING

Connie has multiple risk factors working against her, including her age, her height, having four children, her job, and her weekly bowling. Her greatest risk appears to be her job, which requires heavy work with repetitive bending, twisting, and lifting. Doing a physical job and being out of shape create more risk to Connie because of her lack of muscle strength, flexibility, and overall endurance. In addition, having a vice principal who is constantly yelling during serving time is a potential risk to Connie, since it could disrupt Connie's concentration while working, which might lead to an injury. As a result, Connie scored a risk total of 152.3 points (see Appendix C), putting her at a high risk for back pain. The following back-building techniques were used to help Connie reduce her risk.

Not surprisingly, Connie had recently developed an episode of back pain. After treating her condition and rating her risk, I advised her to make some lifestyle changes because I feared she would again suffer with back pain. After experiencing back pain for the first time, Connie was willing to make changes to help prevent back pain from recurring. Connie was even more encouraged to exercise once she learned her own risk factors for back pain. She could see that if she didn't make some changes, it was likely that she would develop a bad back and possibly experience permanent suffering.

Because of her physical job, Connie began the back-friendly workout to build her strength, flexibility, and endurance. At first, Connie was not thrilled with the idea of having to weight train, and the only conditioning exercise she wanted to participated in was dancing. Years ago, Connie had tried to get her husband Curly to sign up for a disco dancing class with her, but Curly had no desire to do so.

This time, Connie tried a new approach. Knowing that Curly loves country western music, she hoped he might be interested in dancing at a country western dance club. Curly, who never thought of himself as a dancer, was a little reserved about Connie's idea, although he had watched line dancing on TV and always thought it would be fun. Connie also reminded Curly that she wasn't the only one in the household with a physical job. After some thought, Curly, a carpenter and former local football player, liked the idea of getting back into shape and reducing his risk for back pain at the same time. As a result, Connie has not only a dance partner but also someone to keep her motivated to weight train, since Curly has enjoyed weight training ever since he was in high school.

Connie and Curly weight train at the local health club four times a week for about 30 minutes and practice their line dancing three times a week for about an hour. Connie and Curly enjoy dancing so much they now travel once a month to different dance halls with other members of the health club.

Connie has learned how to minimize twisting and forward and backward bending during exercise. Now she is ready to apply these same principles to her work. After reviewing her job duties, I recommended that she seek others' help when possible, use supports and carrying devices, and rotate with fellow workers certain high-risk job activities to minimize the effect of these repetitive movements. Connie was a little resistant to my recommendations because she felt I was just having others do her high-risk chores at their expense.

I reminded Connie that the risk at her job was the improper repetitive movements, which create the wear and tear to the back that leads to pain. If she were to have a student help her lift things at work, these overuse movements would be lessened, while the student would have done very little of these repetitive movements and therefore would not be at risk. With regards to her rotating jobs with her co-workers, she's not necessarily putting them at a higher risk, either. For example, many athletes cross-train to reduce their risk of injury. Athletes tend to use the same muscles over and over in their sport, often creating repetitive overuse injuries (tendinitis, bursitis, back pain, etc.). These athletes thus train using different activities to work opposing muscle groups, not only creating muscle strength and balance but also allowing overworked muscles to rest. This in turn helps to prevent injuries from overuse. Rotating jobs is a form of cross-training that allows one's co-workers to minimize repetitive movements by

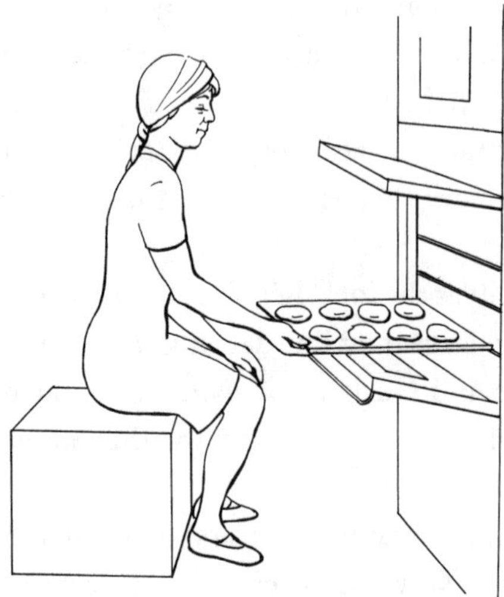

Fig. 6-4. Putting food in oven correctly

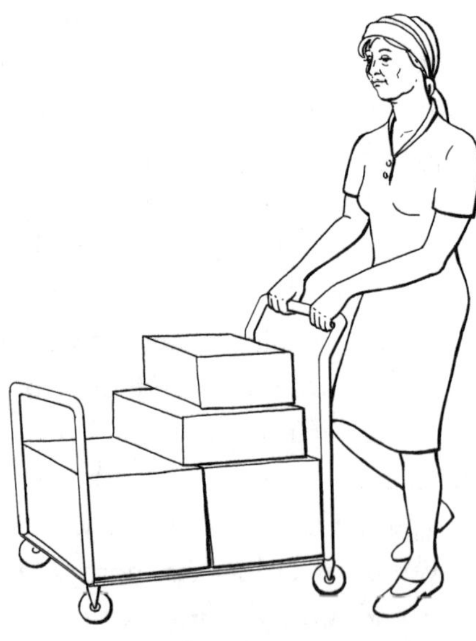

Fig. 6-5. Carting food

using different muscle groups during different job tasks and allowing a rest period to overworked muscle groups.

Connie was now ready to make changes at work. Her first change occurred at delivery time. Instead of having the driver drop off all deliveries at the kitchen, Connie now has him deliver all frozen and dry goods to the building where the freezer and storage room are located. When rotating heavy inventory from the rear to the front, Connie wears a lifting belt to support her back. When stacking the inventory, Connie is careful to maintain a straight back and uses her legs as much as possible when lifting. In addition, she wears her belt when lifting heavy pots or trays.

Connie uses a wooden box to sit on when placing trays into and taking them out of the lower oven or warmer (Fig. 6-4). This prevents her from bending forward and twisting. Connie also uses the wooden box to stand on when placing trays into and taking them out of the upper oven or warmer. This prevents Connie from reaching too far forward. When Connie brings food from the freezer or storage

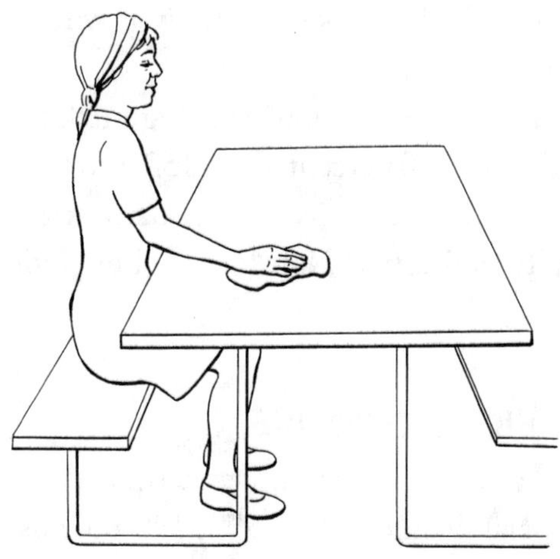

Fig. 6-6. Cleaning table correctly

room, she places it on a cart and transports it to the kitchen instead of carrying the items herself (Fig. 6-5). She also uses the cart to transport food from the kitchen to the serving line.

Connie's fifth-grade student helpers help to rotate the inventory, place food from the freezer and storage room onto the cart, and unload the cart once in the kitchen. The students also transport food that doesn't require heating from the kitchen to the serving line, which has helped to eliminate delays in the serving line. As a result, the vice principal has stopped yelling at Connie and her co-workers.

Connie now cleans the tables sitting down instead of leaning over the benches. When sitting, she is able to clean her side of the table without reaching too far forward (Fig. 6-6). Connie then slides down the bench as she cleans her side of the table before cleaning the other side. After each meal, Connie and two of her co-workers rotate job duties. One cleans the tables the way Connie has recently learned; the other cleans the dishes; a third person helps to prepare the food for the next meal.

Even with these changes, Connie still has a job with a great deal of repetitive bending, twisting, lifting, pushing, and pulling. This is why it is so important that Connie continue to exercise. The back-friendly workout will provide Connie with a full-body approach to improve her conditioning and flexibility and build her muscle strength. The back-friendly workout will also provide Connie with minimal forward and backward bending and twisting when exercising. This will be helpful in preventing an overuse injury that could cause back pain. Being strong and fit the back-friendly way will be Connie's best defense in preventing a bad back.

As a result of these changes, Connie is no longer at high risk for back pain. She has lowered her risk over 60 percent, from 152.3 to 60.5 (See Appendix C). Having made different choices in her daily activities, Connie is now living a healthier lifestyle. Now let's see how Otis can develop a healthier lifestyle.

OTIS THE OFFICE EXECUTIVE

Otis is currently employed as an office executive at B.N. Paine Incorporated as a certified financial planner. He is 5'7", 198 pounds, 52 years old, and presently going through a divorce. He has smoked for the past 20 years.

As a golfer, Otis has won the city championship twice and competes regularly throughout Northern California. As a retirement planner for the employees of B.N. Paine, he is able to schedule his work in the afternoon and evening. This schedule allows him to golf every morning and compete on the weekends.

For the majority of the day, Otis is sitting (Fig. 6-7). Even when golfing, he sits most of the time in his golf cart. Otis has been driving over an hour an half to work for about 20 years and regularly drives one to four hours on the weekend to attend a golf tournament.

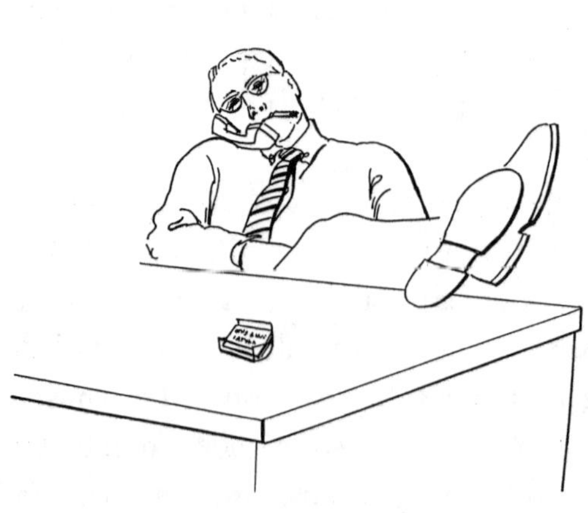

Fig. 6-7. Otis at work

Otis is rarely at home to spend time with his wife and two children. Once a month, he tries to take his teenage son or daughter with him to different tournaments. His children enjoy the traveling and even accompany their father on the golf course as his caddy. For years his wife Olivia hadn't minded being a golf widow, but lately she has grown tired of being left alone and is seeking a divorce.

Even though Otis was at one time a wrestler, he has developed a low tolerance to pain. He therefore has much more anxiety than others about the probability of experiencing pain. In addition, Otis's company is downsizing, and Otis is afraid that either he or his partner will lose his job.

As a large employer who is concerned about rising health care costs, B.N. Paine offers its employees free membership to a local health club. Unfortunately, Otis believes he is too old to start an exercise program. He also feels that weight training might alter his golf swing. Knowing he is unfit, Otis keeps telling himself that he is going to start walking, but he has yet to begin.

BACK BUILDING

Otis can use the following back-building techniques to help him reduce his risk factors for back pain. Otis has nine risk factors working against him: prolonged sitting, golfing, smoking, commuting, his age, and the fact that he is a former wrestler, is overweight and physically out of shape, and has a low pain tolerance. Let's see how Otis can make changes in his lifestyle that will reduce his risk for back pain.

When his golfing partner developed a permanent back disability, Otis began to worry about his own back and overall health. After consulting with Otis, I was able to show him that the best way to reduce his risk for back pain (as well as heart disease) was to exercise and live a healthy lifestyle. I showed him how certain types of exercise could help him to reduce the known risks of back pain.

After receiving an examination and getting the okay to participate in an exercise program, Otis realized that he wasn't too old to start exercising. In fact, exercise will help Otis to remain physically independent in his later years. Otis was surprised to learn how much golf could actually harm his back and elected to choose walking as his conditioning exercise. Initially, Otis refused to give up golf, thinking he would get his walking done on the golf course. Unfortunately, twisting would still occur, and walking with frequent stopping wouldn't be enough to condition his body.

If it hadn't been for the advice of one of his clients, Otis would probably have given up on the thought of exercise. Otis had told his client that he was thinking of starting to exercise. The client had agreed that this made sense, since Otis had always preached to him about thinking long term when investing for his retirement. Otis's client went on to say, "It doesn't make any sense for us to think long term about our investments and not think long term about our health. I mean, what is the point in saving money for our retirement if we aren't going to be around to enjoy it?"

Otis was now ready to make major changes in his lifestyle. His first change was to participate in the back-friendly workout. At first, Otis walked on the treadmill at the company health club. He then switched to the stair-climbing machine and finally decided he preferred the stationary bike.

He weight trained with a fellow employee and did his conditioning either before or after work. Initially, Otis didn't want to weight train because he thought it would make him bigger. Since he was trying to lose weight, he didn't want to add pounds. As with many others, I instructed Otis to keep lifting weights even though at first he would gain a few pounds because his muscles would be getting bigger. Since the muscles burn calories, the bigger the muscles, the more calories a person will burn in the long run. Otis could now see that weight training would play a vital role in his goal of losing weight.

Having a competitive nature, Otis has since participated in a number of organized bicycle rides in the area. Unlike his golfing days, however, during which he competed, he is now just trying to improve his time. Since he enjoys riding his bike with others, he has started a company bike club, where once a month, he and his fellow employees participate in group bike rides throughout the state.

After two years of exercising, Otis has reaped the rewards of being fit while reducing many of his risk factors for back pain. Since he started the back-friendly workout, he has quit golfing, gotten into shape, lost weight, increased his pain tolerance, and developed a healthy attitude, which has led him to seek professional help to stop smoking. He is eating healthfully and uses a back cushion when driving to work. While at work, he breaks up the prolonged sitting by doing some stretching exercises, typically doing one exercise every 30 to 40 minutes (Fig. 6-8).

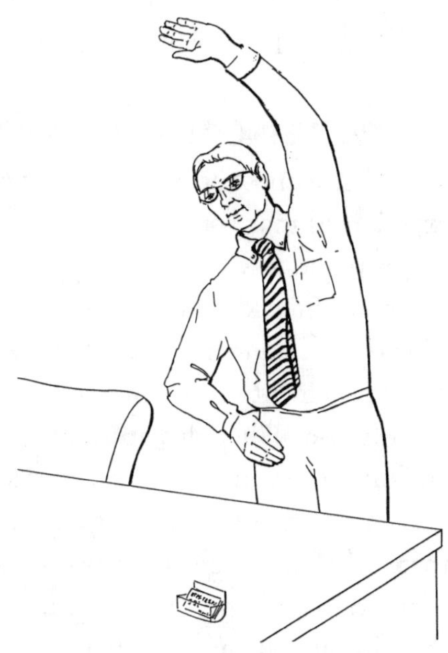

Fig. 6-8. Otis stretching at work

As a result of back building, Otis has lowered his risk total from 141.7 to 34 (see Appendix C), a little over a 75 percent reduction in risk. This reduction in risk lowers Otis from a high-risk category to a more acceptable level. How does Otis feel? Otis will be the first to tell you that two years ago he was an old 52-year-old and today he is a young 54-year-old. Otis obviously feels good about himself and his job and is happy that he is able to spend more time with his children and his wife Olivia, who no longer is a golf widow.

Imagine if Otis had lowered his risk earlier in life, before his exposure to these risk factors could have had a wear-and-tear effect upon his body. But Otis had never been informed regarding his back, and like many people before him, he just assumed he had little control with regards to his own spinal health. Luckily, it wasn't too late for Otis, who hadn't yet developed a back condition causing pain or disability. By lowering his risk, his chances are better that he will not develop back pain or disability in the future.

REFUSING TO GIVE UP YOUR FAVORITE SPORT

Unlike most people, Otis had many significant simultaneous life experiences that encouraged him to make major changes in his life. For example, having his golf partner develop a permanent back disability frightened him. In addition, Otis was embarrassed and felt like a hypocrite asking his clients to think long term so they could improve their retirement years while neglecting to think long term regarding his own overall health status. He had been living a lifestyle that could end his retirement prematurely or lessen his quality of life.

Even with the kind of encouragement that Otis encountered, there will always be those people who refuse to quit their favorite sport. Being a sports enthusiast, I am aware that many people seek their livelihood through their recreational habits. If this is the case with you and you're willing to accept the additional risk, keep doing what you love to do. Simply concentrate on other back-building tools to help prolong your participation in these activities.

Avoiding risky recreational activities isn't your only back-building tool. For example, had Otis continued to play golf and applied other back-building tips to his lifestyle, he still would have dramatically lowered his risk for developing back pain. If Otis had continued to ride a stationary bike and work out the back-friendly way and apply the other back-building tips mentioned earlier while still playing golf, his risk total would be 63, a 55 percent reduction in risk from his original risk total of 141 points.

TAKING CONTROL

No pill or treatment has more of an effect toward maintaining good health than living a healthy lifestyle. As you can see with Connie and Otis, by changing your lifestyle and minimizing certain health risks, you can have some control over your well-being. Most people are aware that if they eat a high-fat diet, smoke, and don't regularly exercise, they are putting themselves at risk for heart disease. Unfortunately, most people aren't aware of the multiple risk factors for back pain. As a result, this is a leading cause of disability. The more you work to eliminate these risk factors, the better your chances of preventing back pain and disability.

You need to take control of your health. Why suffer from your own abuse and neglect? A bad back can leave you with permanent pain and disability. Start exercising today! Exercise not only is the most comprehensive form of any preventive approach for back pain but also can help you feel good about your body both physically and mentally. In addition, your overall health will improve. Join others who have found exercise to be energizing and fun. If Connie and Otis can exercise and use other back-building techniques, so can you.

The following chapters present the back-friendly workout. Chapter 7 covers the warming-up and cooling-down processes, Chapters 8 and 9 discuss conditioning, and Chapter 10 presents information on weight training. Unlike others, this is the ONLY COMPLETE EXERCISE PROGRAM designed to minimize or eliminate all categories of the known risk factors of back pain.

CHAPTER 7

Warming Up and Cooling Down

ISN'T IT CURIOUS that people in developed countries tend to suffer from insufficient movement and a lack of a variety of movements. This sedentary lifestyle creates muscle imbalances within the body. Research in Europe has found that certain unused muscles tend to remain tight among sedentary individuals, while other neglected muscles tend to weaken. Table 7-1 lists muscles that tend to tighten and weaken from disuse and misuse.

These researchers found that it is important to stretch the tight muscles before trying to strengthen the weak muscles. Normally, there is a balance among many opposing muscle groups, although imbalances can occur, creating certain tight muscles to weaken opposing muscles. For example, tight back muscles will weaken the abdominal muscles. When stretching tight muscles, your body will in a reflex fashion simultaneously strengthen the opposing weaker muscles while relaxing the tight muscles. It has been theorized that strengthening weak muscles without first stretching tight muscles will further compound this muscle imbalance. It is therefore essential to always stretch

TABLE 7-1

LOCATION OF SOME MUSCLE GROUPS THAT TEND TO TIGHTEN OR WEAKEN

Tighten	Weaken
Upper Body	Upper Body
back of the arms	abdominals muscles
chest	mid-back muscles
upper-back muscles	shoulders
low-back muscles	
front of the neck	
oblique stomach muscles	
Lower Body	Lower Body
inner thighs	front thigh muscles
hip flexor muscles	
back of the thighs	

before and after exercising. This is significant when you consider that these changes alter normal posture and play an important role in the development of many painful conditions.

The importance of stretching is shared by the American College of Sports Medicine, which states the following in it's guidelines for exercise:

> *Stretching can aid in improving and maintaining range of motion in a joint or series of joints. Of particular concern is maintenance of flexibility in the lower back and the back thigh region. Lack of flexibility in these regions is associated with the increased risk for development of chronic lower back pain. Therefore, preventive exercise programs should include activities that promote maintenance of good flexibility, particularly in the lower back.*

Stretching plays a vital role not only in your warm-up routine but also in the maintenance of a healthy back. By doing your warm-up routine before any exercise, your body will achieve a sufficient variety of movements that will help to maintain normal muscle balance while preparing your body for your exercise workout.

Increasing the body's muscle temperature reduces stiffness from exercise by increasing range of motion in the joints and muscles. Warm-up apparently leads to a more efficient contraction among the muscles, thereby improving athletic performance and possibly preventing muscle injury.

The following guidelines must be met for a fully effective warm-up:

1. Raise your body temperature one or two degrees, even to the point where you begin to sweat.
2. Do some specific movements related to the type of exercise you will be performing as well as some general body movements.
3. If you are a well-conditioned individual, you will require a longer warm-up (20-30 minutes) than a sedentary individual (5-15 minutes).
4. Always include stretching to develop or maintain adequate flexibility.
5. Quit your warm-up a few minutes before you start exercising.

WARM-UP ROUTINE

Of the four components of exercise (flexibility, conditioning, muscle strengthening, and muscle endurance), flexibility is usually the least performed. During stretching, a number of movements are usually at risk for developing back pain. Therefore, when you warm up before the conditioning and weight-training phases of exercise, try to eliminate as much twisting, arching, and forward bending of your back as possible.

Your warm-up routine will differ depending on the type of workout you are preparing yourself for. If you're warming up before a conditioning workout such as swimming, walking, or cycling, start your routine doing those exercises. These conditioning exercises should be done at a slow pace for approximately five to ten minutes, depending on your fitness level. You're then ready for the stretching phase of your warm-up.

If you're warming up before weight training or any nonconditioning activity, you must supplement your warm-up with some type of conditioning activity to increase your heart rate and raise your body temperature. For example, before weight training, use the treadmill, stair climber, or cycling machine at your health club, again at a slow pace for approximately five to ten minutes. If you are doing a nonconditioning recreational activity such as softball, try jogging around the field for your warm-up before stretching.

Now you are ready to do your stretching exercises. When stretching, pay special attention to the technique of the exercise. It is important to hold each stretch, with no jerky or bouncing movements. In other words, stretch gradually and hold (no bouncing) when you feel mild tension, not pain. If one side is more restricted than the other, always do the tighter side first. Bouncing or jerking while stretching could cause tearing of the muscles or joints, creating an injury.

STRETCHING EXERCISES

The following exercises are to be done in the sequence as listed. Start by lying down, then move to the standing position. You will need a belt or rope for three of the stretching exercises. I recommend purchasing a seat belt because they're durable and inexpensive. It is best to stretch on a carpeted or padded area. Spend about 15 seconds on each stretching exercise. Breathe calmly and do not hold your breath when stretching. Never stretch if you think you have a torn muscle or any muscle injury without first consulting with your doctor. Remember, stretching too hard can cause muscle soreness, so easy does it. Depending on your fitness level, your warm-up will take approximately 15-20 minutes.

1. Mid-back

This stretch works primarily the upper to mid-back and certain arm muscles. Lie flat on your back and straighten your arms above your

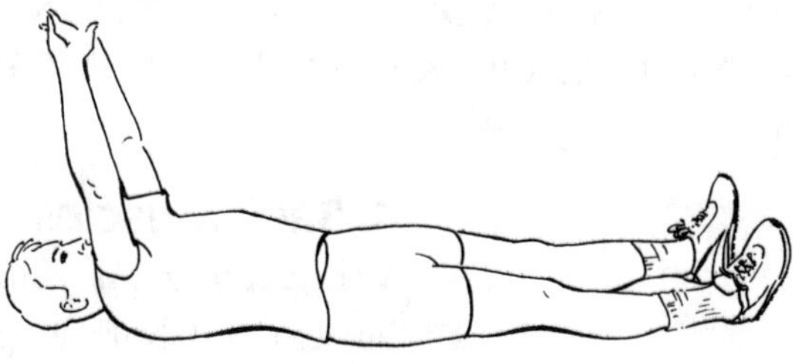

Fig. 7-1. Mid-back

shoulders, lifting arms upward (Fig. 7-1). Stretch as far as possible or to the point of tension and hold for 15 seconds.

2. Back of the thigh

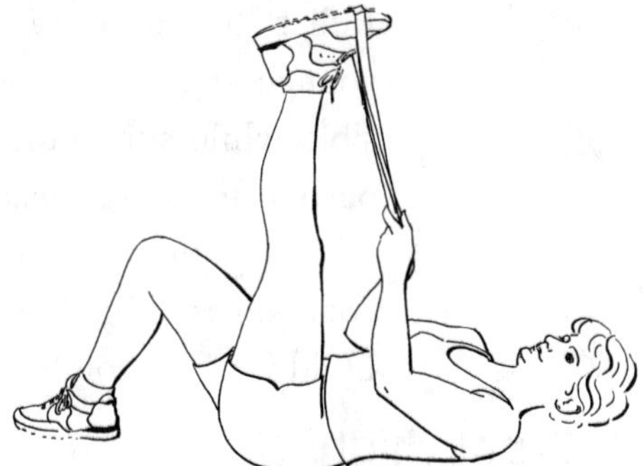

Fig. 7-2. Back of the thigh

Lie flat on your back with one knee bent and the opposite leg straight. Using a belt or rope wrapped around your foot, lift the straight leg to the point of tolerance (Fig. 7-2) and hold for 15 seconds. Then lower your leg to surface. Do the same with opposite leg.

3. Buttocks/low back

While lying on your back with one leg bent, grip your hands behind your lower thigh of the opposite leg above the knee. Pull the thigh toward your chest while keeping your head on the floor (Fig. 7-3). Hold this position for 15 seconds.

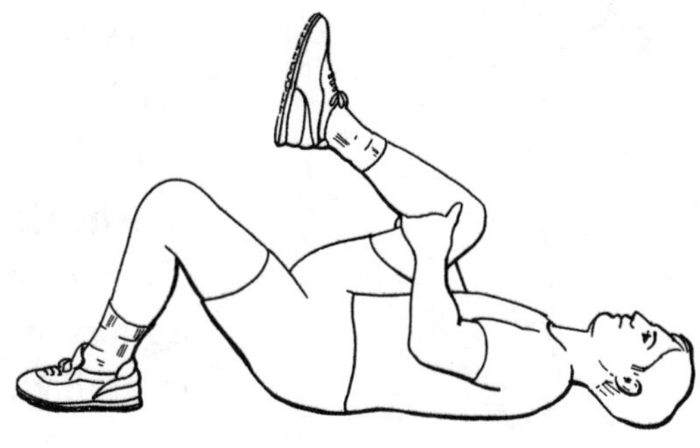

Fig. 7-3. Buttocks/low back

Repeat with other leg. ALWAYS GRIP YOUR HANDS AROUND YOUR THIGH AND NOT AROUND YOUR KNEE OR LOWER LEG.

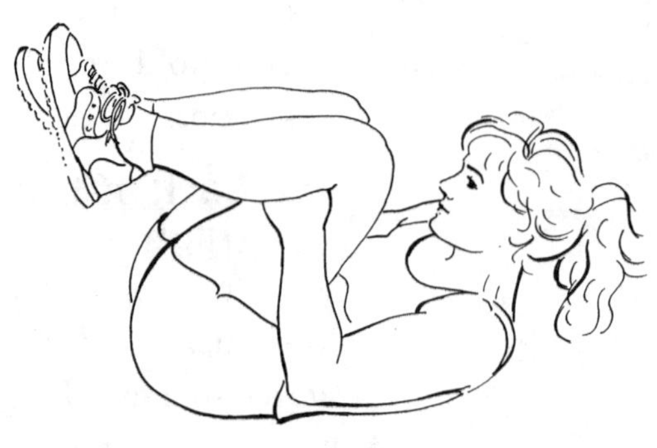

Fig. 7-4. Back muscles

4. Back muscles

While lying on your back, bend both legs and grip your hands behind your thighs. Pull both legs toward your chest as far as possible while simultaneously lifting your head off the ground toward your knees (Fig. 7-4). Hold for 15 seconds.

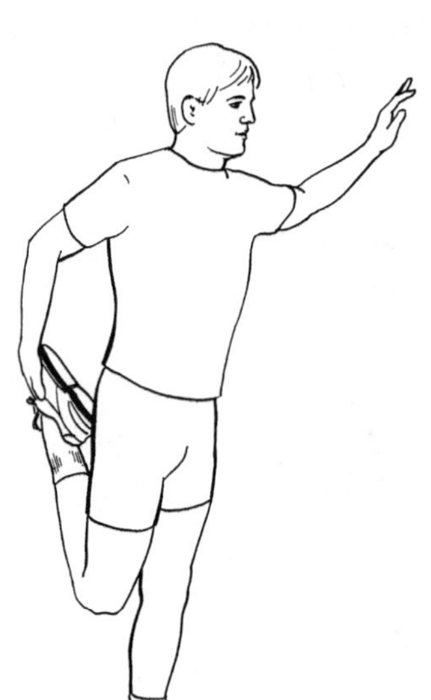

Fig. 7-5. Front thigh

5. Front thigh

From the standing position bend your knee and grab your foot (Fig. 7-5). Pull your foot toward your buttocks. Hold at the point of tension for 15 seconds, then repeat with other leg. If necessary, lean against the wall with opposite hand to help maintain your balance.

6. Hip flexors

From a standing position, lunge one leg forward. Rest your hands on your front thigh (Fig. 7-6). To get the best stretch of the hip flexors, make sure your knee is not in front of your ankle or bent more than 90 degrees. To prevent a knee injury, bend knee only about a third of its normal motion. Move hip forward, keeping your back straight at all times and toes pointing forward. Hold at the point

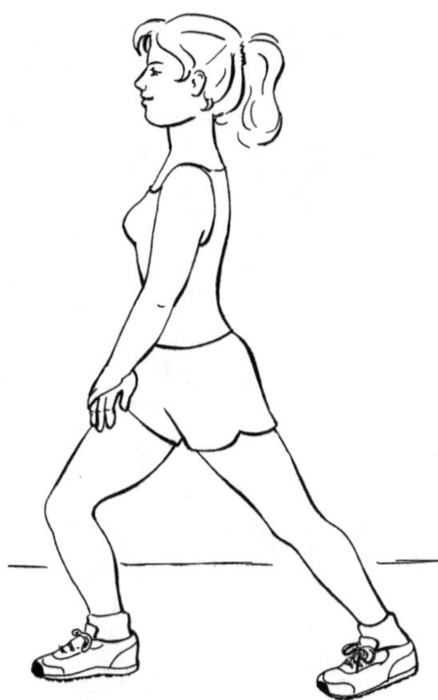

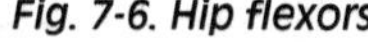

Fig. 7-6. Hip flexors

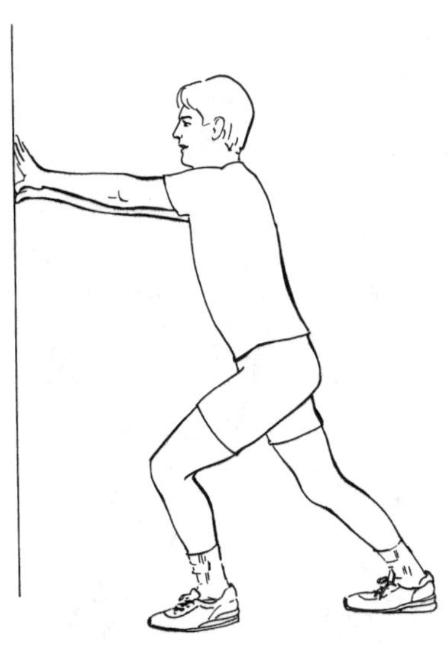

Fig. 7-7. Calf (lower leg)

of tension for 15 seconds, then repeat with the other leg.

7. Calf muscles

Standing with one foot in front of the other, lean your straight body forward, with your hands placed against a wall (Fig. 7-7). Move your hips forward to the point of tension in the rear lower leg and hold for 15 seconds. Make sure toes are always pointing forward. Repeat with other leg.

8. Inner thigh

From a standing position, straddle your legs sideways. With the supporting leg bent, slide out other leg, keeping it straight (Fig. 7-8). Keep your

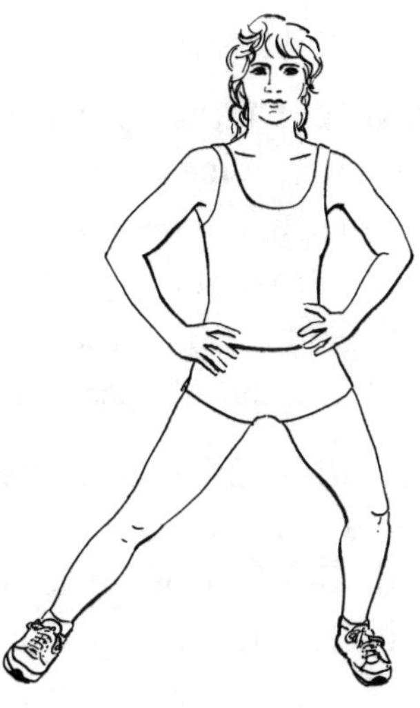

Fig. 7-8. Inner thigh

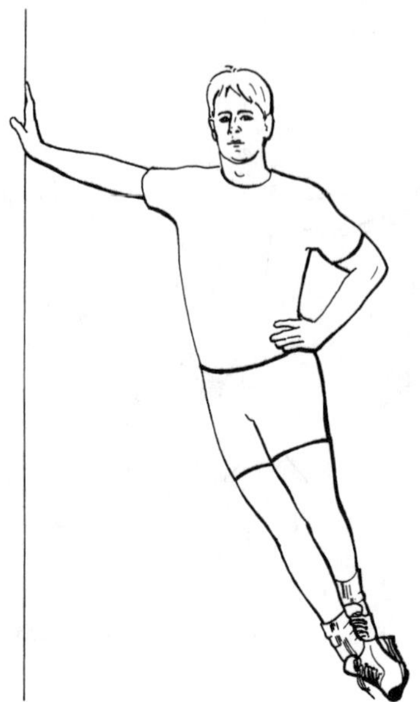

Fig. 7-9. Outer thigh and hips

Fig. 7-10. Back and rib cage

back straight at all times. Once you feel tension in the inner thigh, hold for 15 seconds, then repeat with other leg.

9. Outer thigh and hip

From a standing position, lean your body sideways, with your arm supporting your upper body against the wall. Place your foot nearest the wall in front of other foot (Fig. 7-9). Place opposite arm at the waist and bend the hip area toward the wall. Hold at the point of tension for 15 seconds. Repeat other side.

10. Back and ribcage muscles

Stand with your feet shoulder width apart. Lift one arm over your head in the direction of the side bending. Place opposite hand on your waist while you stretch (Fig. 7-10). Bend slowly to the point of tension, then hold stretch for 15 seconds. Do not bend your knees. For further stretch, breathe out when bending sideways. When through, slowly return to starting position. Repeat other side.

11. Upper back and front of arms

Stand with your feet shoulder width apart. Raise both arms above your head and join hands with your palms facing upward (Fig. 7-11). Keep your chin level while holding at the point of tension for 15 seconds.

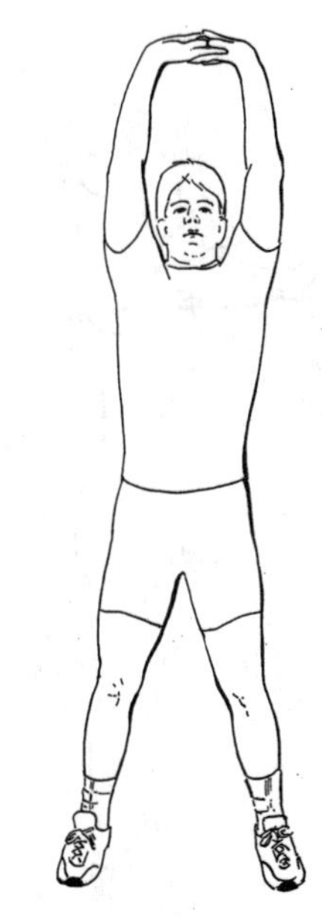

Fig. 7-11. Upper back and front of arms

12. Upper back, back of the upper arm, and shoulders

In a standing position, reach behind your head with one arm with your hand (palm down) reaching as far down the center of your back as possible. Reach the opposite arm behind your mid-back with your hand (palm facing outward) reaching up to other hand. Grab fingers and hold (Fig. 7-12). Repeat with opposite arms. If possible, grab fingers and pull together and hold for 15 seconds. This stretch has been used to determine upper-body flexibility. Unfortunately, many (especially those who lift weights) will not be able to do the above stretch. For those who cannot, don't give up hope; there

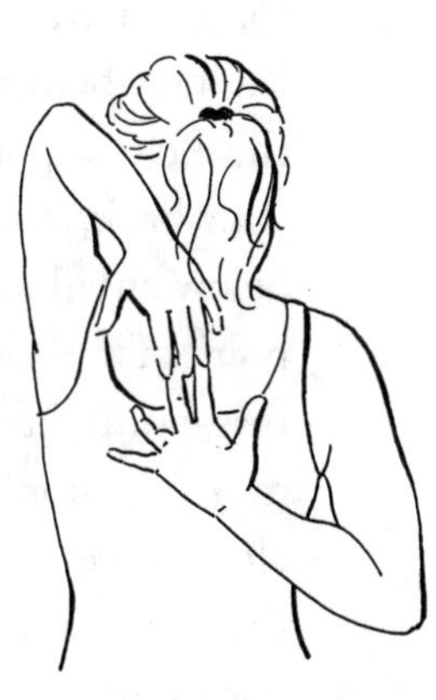

Fig. 7-12. Upper back/back of arms/shoulders

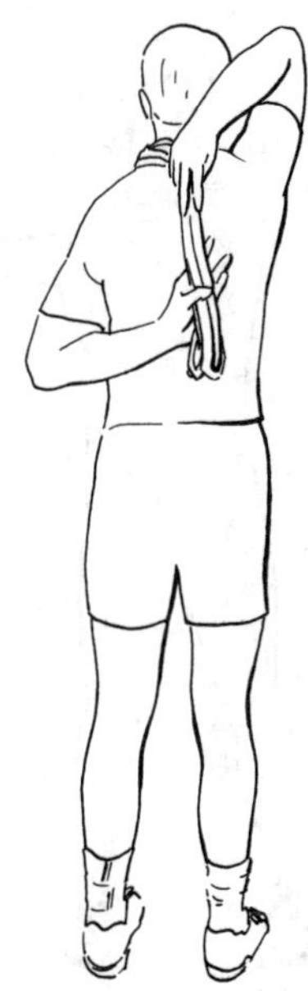

Fig. 7-13. 7-12 done with belt

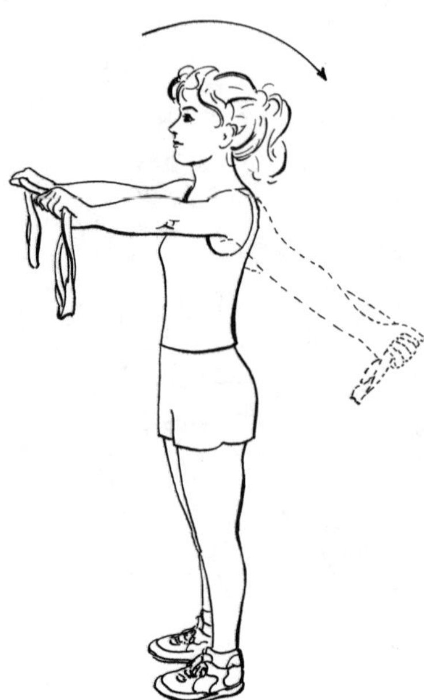

Fig. 7-14. Chest

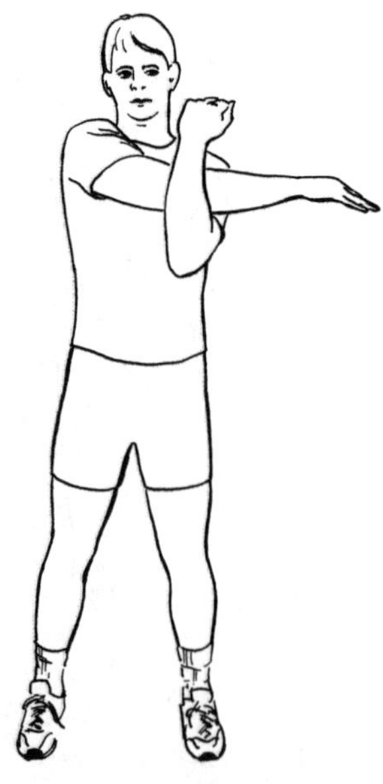

Fig. 7-15. Shoulder

is an alternate technique. Hold a belt or folded towel behind your head with the upper arm; with the lower arm, reach up and hold onto the belt (Fig. 7-13). Slowly move your hands closer together on the belt to the point of tension. Hold for 15 seconds, then repeat with opposite arms.

13. Chest muscles

In a standing position while holding a belt or folded towel with both hands, straighten arms and pull belt or towel up and over your head and behind your back (Fig. 7-14). Make sure to keep your eyes focused straight ahead so that you don't drop your head. If you can't raise the belt up and over your head, your hands might be too close together on the belt. If so, get a wider grip. Never force the belt behind your back. Once the belt is placed gently behind your back, keep your hands at or below shoulder level. Hold at the point of tension for 15 seconds. At this point, if you wish to apply more tension, move your hands closer together on the belt. When through with stretch, simply release the grip on one side of the belt.

14. Shoulders

In a standing position, with one arm pull the other arm across your chest toward the opposite shoulder (Fig. 7-15). Hold for 15 seconds and then repeat with other arm.

15. Neck muscles

Tilt your head toward your left shoulder and hold at point of tension for 15 seconds (Fig. 7-16). Again tilt your head, this time toward your right shoulder, and hold for 15 seconds.

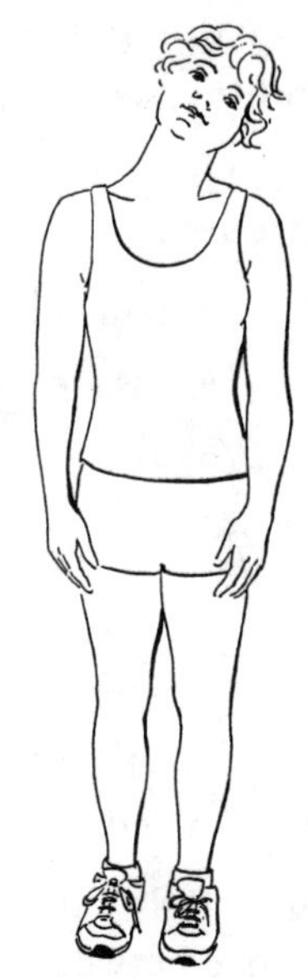

Fig. 7-16. Side of neck

Slowly tilt your head backward as far as possible and hold for 15 seconds (Fig. 7-17), making sure to hold onto a supporting structure to help prevent you from losing your balance. Finally, drop your head forward as far as possible, placing your chin on your chest, and hold for 15 seconds (Fig. 7-18).

A word of caution when tilting your head backwards to stretch neck. Don't tilt head backwards and turn your head to the left or right at the same time. In extremely rare circumstances this has been known to cause a stroke. These combined movements have

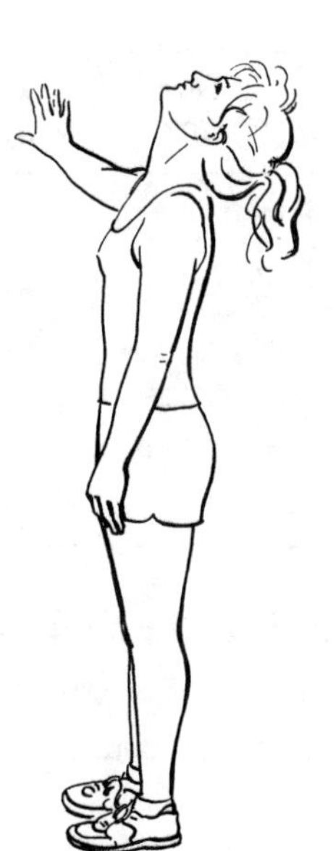

Fig. 7-17. Front of neck

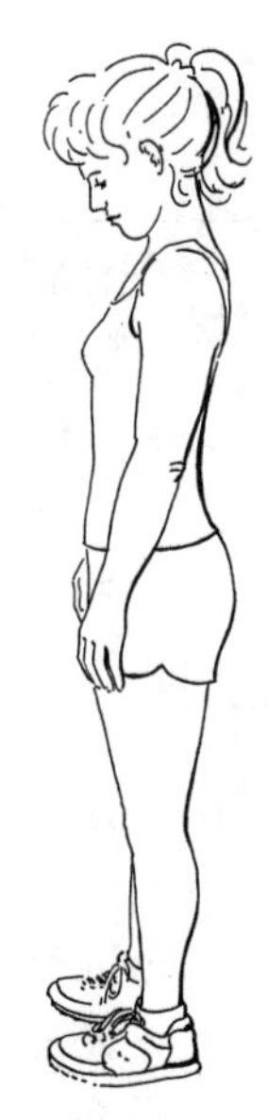

Fig. 7-18. Back of neck

resulted in pinching or tearing of the neck arteries, developing stroke conditions.

The following daily activities which include the above neck movements, have been reported to cause a stroke.

Certain calisthenics	Driving a motor vehicle
Tennis (serving)	Sneeze/coughing
Yoga	Hair washing at beauty salons

COOL-DOWN ROUTINE

A cool-down routine is an important component of an exercise program. Although there is some debate about whether a cool-down helps to reduce soreness, it still can serve as an additional way to improve back flexibility, prevent muscle injury, and help to maintain balance between opposing muscle groups.

A cool-down routine typically is not as long as a warm-up routine. Only six of the fifteen warm-up exercises are recommended (Table 7-2):

TABLE 7-2

COOL-DOWN ROUTINE

1. Back of the thigh (Fig. 7-2)
2. Back muscles (Fig. 7-4)
3. Hip flexors (Fig. 7-6)
4. Back and ribcage muscles (Fig. 7- 10)
5. Chest muscles (Fig. 7-14)
6. Neck muscles (Fig. 7-16, 7-17, 7-18)

You may be wondering why stretching the back of your thighs, hip flexors, and chest muscles is important to back flexibility. As shown earlier, these groups are usually tight and hamper back flexibility in several ways.

Having the back of the thigh muscles flexible will help in proper bending and lifting. A proper way to bend forward is to bend at your hips while keeping your back straight (Fig. 7-19). Having flexible back-of-thigh muscles allows the back to be positioned the same as if you were standing. Incorrect forward bending (Fig. 7-20), where your back is rounded, applies undue stress upon your discs, joints, and ligaments.

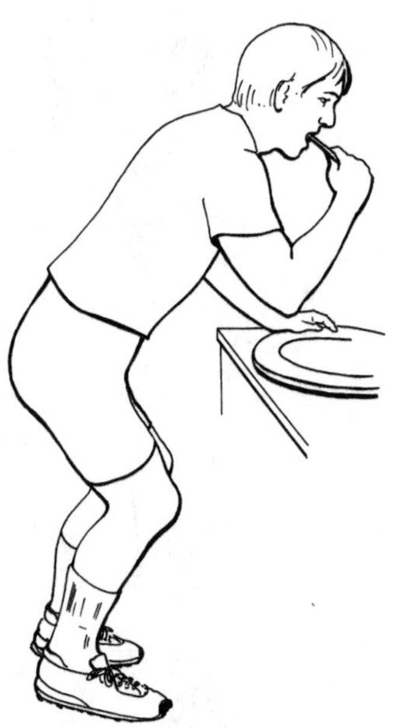

Fig. 7-19. Flexible thighs upon bending

It is best to try to eliminate forward bending, although there are times when you will be left with no choice but to bend. At these times, you should practice proper forward bending, such as when leaning over a sink to brush your teeth or when lifting something out of your car trunk. Having flexible muscles is essential for this type of forward bending.

The hip flexor muscles begin on the low-back vertebrae and attach to the thigh bone directly below the hip. These muscles are important for maintaining erect posture. Tight or underdeveloped hip flexor muscles can create problems for your back. Tight hip flexor muscles can create an increased forward curve in the low back (Fig. 7-21). This increased curve, commonly called swayback, not only alters normal mechanics of the low back but also puts excessive strain upon the joints and discs. Swayback is

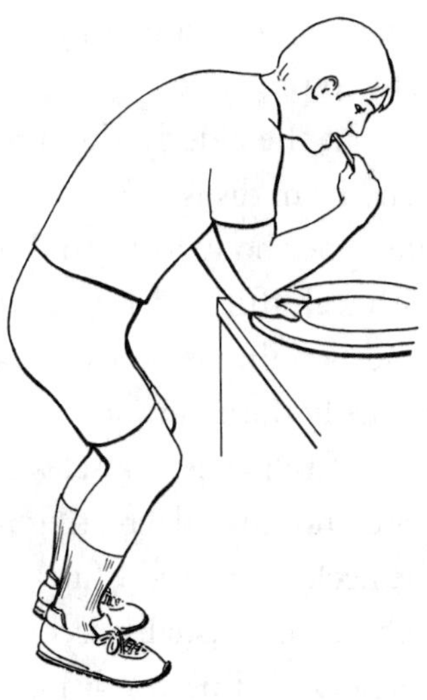

Fig. 7-20. Inflexible thighs upon bending

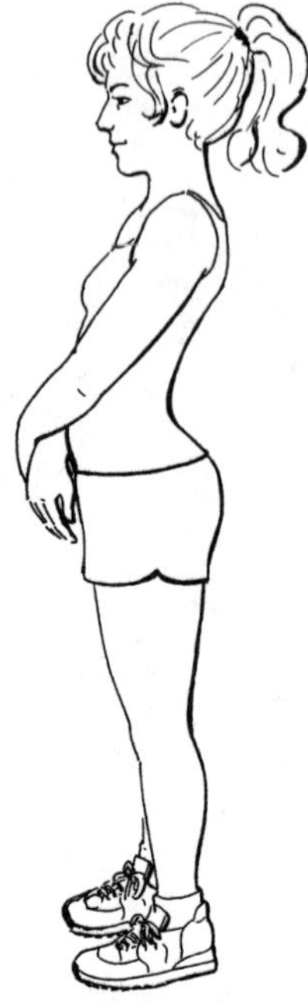

Fig. 7-21. Swayback

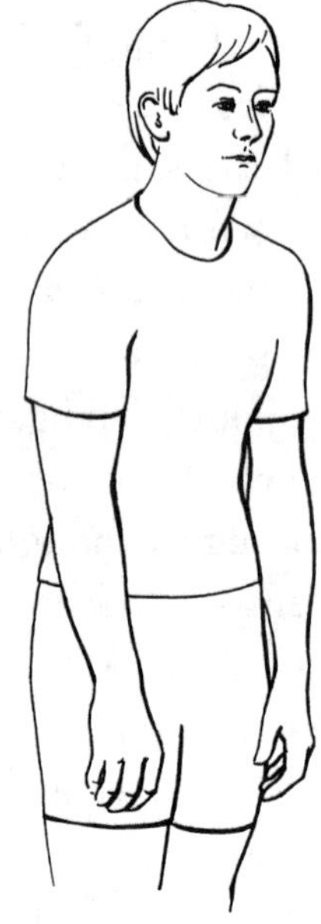

Fig. 7-22. Effects of tight chest muscles

usually accompanied by weak abdominal muscles, which allow the belly to protrude.

In the elderly, the hip flexor muscles shrink and lose their elasticity from disuse. As a result, these muscles become smaller and pull the upper body forward. You may have seen this in elderly who walk with a shuffle and lean their upper body forward. This constant forward bending is detrimental to the back, especially at this age when typically there is more wear and tear present in the spine.

If the chest muscles are tight, they will pull the shoulders forward and inward, creating rounded shoulders (Fig. 7-22). This causes the neck to protrude, further compounding the problem. This postural imbalance is usually accompanied by weak upper back muscles. Left unchecked, this condition can lead to further strain and thus more wear and tear upon the neck and upper back regions.

SUMMARY

These warm-up and cool-down routines will prepare both your back and your body for your conditioning and strengthening routines. Without these warm-up and cool-down routines, you are putting yourself at risk for injury. Regarding your back, warm-up/cool-down routines are essential for developing and maintaining muscle balance, a critical component in achieving and maintaining a healthy back.

For more information on stretching, see the recommended reading list in appendix A. These books can provide you with other stretching procedures that might be related to your specific conditioning exercise.

CHAPTER 8

Conditioning

THE CONDITIONING PART of your workout involves an activity that will increase your breathing, get your heart pumping harder, and probably make you perspire. When done correctly, conditioning activities will improve your heart, your lungs, the shape of your body, and, of course, your back.

Excessive weight around your midsection will place some risk to your low back. Having a pot belly alters the normal mechanics of your back by shifting your center of gravity forward. This shift in weight bearing places more physical stress upon your back and may lead to repetitive wear and tear within your spine. Unlike stretching and weight training, conditioning is the primary part of an exercise program that will help to burn off body fat.

To determine your proper weight, see the height-to-weight chart (in Appendix B). Your actual amount of body fat can be best measured by underwater weighing. Judging your fat content by looking in the mirror is not a good idea, since it is possible to be thin and have a high body fat level. Check with your local health club to find where you can get your body fat measured.

Even if you exercise regularly, you will still lose some muscle as you grow older. Since this loss of muscle will increase your tendency to gain body fat as you age, every 15 years after age 20 you'll need to add one percent to your normal range of body fat until age 65. As a result, the maximum normal body fat for men is between 15 percent and 18 percent, while the women's maximum is between 25 percent and 28 percent. It is best to keep your fat content at the mid to lower range (see Table 8-1) when you are young. As you will learn, this will be beneficial as you age, since it's harder to maintain your normal body fat as you grow older. Generally, obesity is indicated at greater than 25 percent and 30 percent body fat for men and women, repectively.

TABLE 8-1

NORMAL RANGE OF BODY FAT

Men		Women	
Ages		Ages	
20-34	10%-15%	20-34	20%-25%
35-49	11%-16%	35-49	21%-26%
50-64	12%-17%	50-64	22%-27%
65 & up	13%-18%	65 & up	23%-28%

HOW TO LOSE BODY FAT

A lean person has less risk than an overweight individual for back pain, heart disease, diabetes, and high blood pressure. If that isn't enough motivation to maintain your ideal weight, think about the following. The average American is 20 percent above his or her ideal weight. Yet Americans of comparable age and height who maintain their proper weight tend to live the longest of all Americans. In other words, people of normal weight tend to live longer and are healthier.

At some point in our lives, most of us will gain weight (I personally gained and lost 25 lbs. after graduating from college). You will therefore need to know how to lose weight the correct way. Conditioning exercises help to increase muscle endurance. The higher your fitness level, the more able your body is to provide oxygen and eliminate waste to and from your muscles. Therefore, your muscles are able to go longer without tiring. Since your muscles need oxygen to burn fat, conditioning will improve your ability to use this stored form of energy for fuel. Conditioning done at a low to moderate intensity has been shown to be the best level for fat burning because your body will use the highest amount of oxygen at this level.

Our ability to use oxygen is essential for fat burning. If you elect not to stay fit, you'll lose about two percent per year in your ability to maximally intake oxygen as you age. If as an adult you participate regularly in a conditioning exercise, you will lose only two thirds of one percent per year as you grow older. This difference over the years can be significant in your ability to burn fat as you age. It is thus possible for a 70-year-old person who has stayed fit his or her entire adult life to have the same ability to intake oxygen as an unfit 35-year-old who has been out of shape his or her entire adult life. In addition, the fit 70-year-old would be able to use this amount of oxygen more efficiently than the unfit 35-year-old, thereby making it easier for the 70-year-old to burn fat than the 35-year-old.

If you're concerned about losing fat, you don't want to train at a competitive level. It is best for competitive athletes to lose weight in the off-season so that they can remain competitive. Instead of training at a high intensity, train at a lower intensity for a longer period of time. This way, the average person will be able to increase his or her fitness level and exercise at a level that is optimal for burning fat.

EATING PROPERLY AND CONDITIONING

There are reasons for exercising while trying to lose weight. If you are only eating fewer calories and not exercising, your body may start to break down muscle as a source of energy. Since your muscles burn fat, you're doing your body more harm than good. Following a healthy diet and participating in a complete exercise program will allow you to burn energy efficiently while maintaining (if not increasing the size of) your muscle tissue. In addition, dieting does not increase the amount of calories you burn; exercise does. For example,

Tour De France cyclists will burn approximately 5,900 calories a day, compared to the average 170-pound man, who burns approximately 2,400 calories a day.

Food is broken down into carbohydrates (breads, cereals, fruits, vegetables), protein (beans, dairy products, nuts, meats) and fats (dairy products, meats, oil, nuts, and some vegetables). The key to proper eating is to have a correct balance of these food categories. The American Dietetic Association (ADA) recommends that these different types of food be consumed in the following way. Up to 63 percent of your diet should be carbohydrates, 12 percent to 15 percent of your intake should be protein, and not more than 25 percent of your food consumption should be from fat.

It is also recommended that if you train hard on successive days or compete in endurance activities, you should have a diet in which 65 percent to 70 percent of your total calories come from carbohydrates. At the same time, you will have a 5 percent to 10 percent reduction in calories from consumption of fats. This will allow the body to easily store and digest the extra energy needed for such activities. During what is commonly called carbo loading, a person might eat spaghetti or other foods high in carbohydrates the night before an athletic event.

In regards to fluid intake while exercising, the ADA recommends for the moderate-level exerciser in a moderate climate to consume only water. If the exerciser works at an exhaustive level or in extreme weather conditions, a low dose of a sport beverage is allowed. Ultra-endurance athletes will need a large dose of a sport beverage to enhance their performance.

Eating the correct foods is only part of a proper diet. Without adequate exercise, eating in excess will eventually lead to an increase in body fat. Just because you eat the right types of food doesn't mean you can't gain body fat. The trick is to balance the amount of calories consumed to the amount burned. If your goal is to lose weight, you should slightly alter your intake and the amount of calories you burn. For example, cycling for 30 minutes three times a week can burn approximately 250 calories. You might also want to switch from eating ice cream to having a low-calorie dessert, thus reducing your intake by another 250 calories a week. Since you have to burn 3,500 calories to lose one pound, you can lose a pound approximately every two months with the above changes in exercise and diet. This may sound trivial compared to a rapid-weight-loss program, which could result in your losing 15 pounds in one month. Yet, would you rather lose 15 pounds in one month and feel deprived and risk your health and probably set yourself up to regain the lost weight (and even more) or lose a pound every two months while feeling healthier and satisfied and most likely keeping the weight off? By having it easier to lose weight, you're more likely to stay with your weight-loss program. Exercising will also help you to keep the weight off, which is usually not the case with rapid weight loss.

Unfortunately, some people will feel that if a little alteration in diet and exercise is good, a lot is even better. Many individuals who have decided to lose weight start by going on a low-calorie diet and drastically increase their activity level. This not only is hard to do but also can be a shock to the heart and body, leading to a serious health condition.

CONSEQUENCES OF A POOR DIET

A couple of health conditions can lead to back pain as a result of a poor diet. Rarely found today, osteomalacia, a vitamin D deficiency, can cause weakness and shortening of the vertebrae in adults. More common is osteoporosis, often called brittle bone disease, since the bones become easily broken or fractured. Nearly one third of women in the United States will develop osteoporosis by age 65. By the age of 70, two of every five American women experience a fracture due to osteoporosis. These fractures often occur in the spine, creating pain and permanent impairment.

Osteoporosis in women is commonly believed to be caused by a lack of estrogen and calcium, although low-calcium-consuming cultures found in Singapore and Hong Kong have one tenth to one third the rate of incidence compared to high-calcium-consuming countries, such as the United States and New Zealand. Recent evidence suggests that a high-protein diet, large amounts of caffeine (four or more cups of coffee per day), smoking, the lack of intake of all the different minerals and vitamins (or lack of a balanced diet as recommended above), and the lack of exercise are all related in the development of osteoporosis.

CONDITIONING EXERCISES

As stated earlier, some recreational activities and certain body movements are at risk for developing back pain. These activities and movements should be eliminated from your conditioning phase of exercise. The following activities are recommended, since they have the least amount of twisting, forward bending, and back bending while still providing the potential to work the heart and lungs enough to be classified as a conditioning exercise. Since some of the exercises are better than others, they are rated on a scale of one to ten, with ten being the best (Table 8-2). These ratings are based upon my review of the scientific literature and professional experience as both a physical educator and chiropractor.

TABLE 8-2
EXERCISE RATINGS

Exercise	Rating	Rating	Exercise
Stair climbing	10	9	Water exercise
Walking	10	8	Soccer
Swimming	10	8	Basketball
Stationary bike	9	8	Aerobic dancing
Rope skipping	9	10	Tap dancing

Stair Climbing

Using a stair-climbing machine is highly recommended (Fig. 8-1). You can use this machine at a health club or at home while watching your favorite TV show. Some stair-climbing machines have graded levels of workouts that can challenge the fit individual. Proper technique includes the upright posture with your toes facing forward (not in or out). It is common for individuals as they become tired to lean their upper body forward and rest their arms upon the handrails. Resist this temptation and maintain an upright posture. Your back will appreciate it.

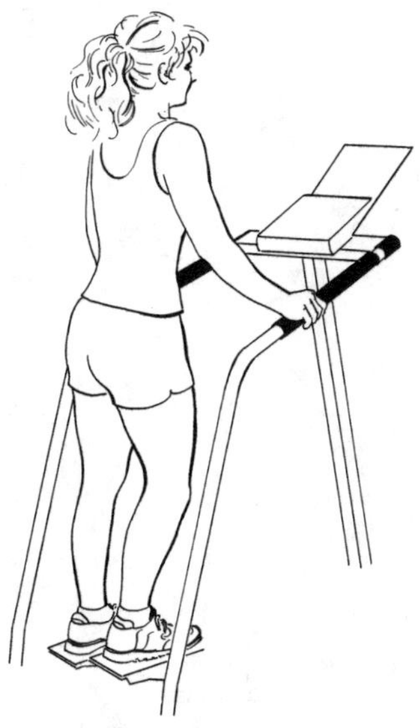

Fig. 8-1. Stair-climbing machine

Stair climbing and cycling are conditioning exercises that primarily use the front thigh muscles. Strength and endurance of these thigh muscles are extremely important for lifting objects properly and maintaining good posture. When these front thigh muscles tire from lifting, you are more likely to bend forward when lifting an object (Fig. 8-2) than to squat and use your legs. Therefore, stair climbing and cycling can be helpful for the person whose job or hobby requires frequent lifting of objects from the floor. (Stair-climbing machines are rated a 10.)

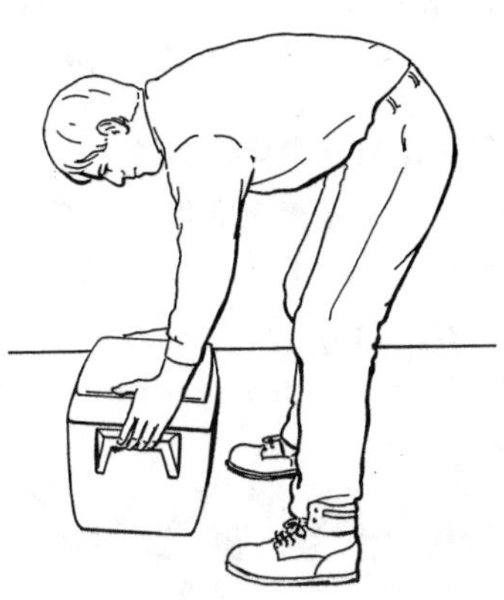

Fig. 8-2. Effects of weak thigh muscles

Walking

Walking is a safe, inexpensive, and convenient way to condition your body (Fig. 8-3). This should be the conditioning exercise of choice for the elderly or for those who have never exercised. Since body fat is burned best during a low to moderate intensity level, walking can help you to lose weight and keep it off. In fact, walking

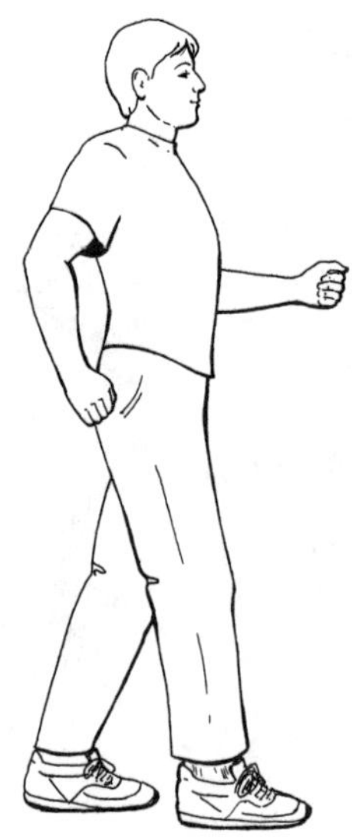
Fig. 8-3. Walking

burns approximately the same amount of calories per mile as jogging. Walking doesn't pound your body as does jogging, although both jogging and walking will tighten the back thigh muscles. Some experts feel that when these muscles remain tight, back pain can result. Therefore, be sure to stretch these muscles well during your warm-up and cool-down routines. Another disadvantage of walking is that it takes longer to get a conditioning effect than it does from other activities, such as stair climbing or cycling. To get a conditioning effect, you will need to walk at a steady and rapid pace—no strolling. Your breathing should be relaxed, and you should use vigorous arm and leg movements. You should wear a good pair of walking shoes to help prevent injury. Heel-to-toe landing of the feet is advised, with toes pointing forward, not in or out. (Walking is rated a 10.)

Swimming

Swimming is a unique form of exercise in that there is little gravitation load placed upon your back, since your weight is supported by water (Fig. 8-4). This is helpful for overweight people, who might otherwise develop injuries by overloading their muscles and joints. The butterfly stroke should be avoided, since it involves tremendous forward and backward bending of the spine. Some swimmers develop back pain while doing

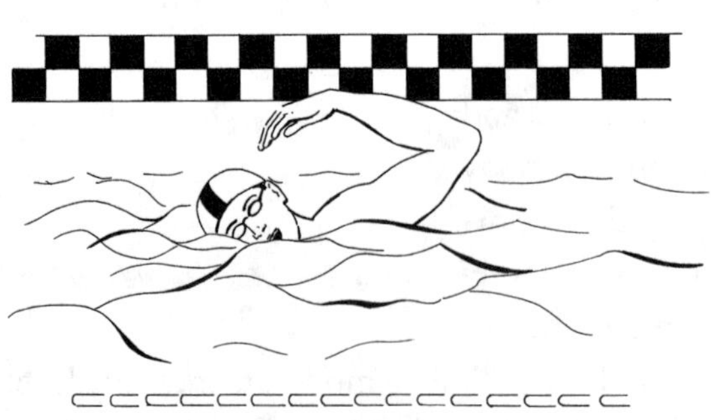
Fig. 8-4. Swimming

the crawl or the breaststroke. If pain develops, it's best to alternate these strokes with the sidestroke or backstroke. When swimming the crawl, make sure to alternate your breathing from side to side. This way you don't consistently turn your head to one side to breathe, which could lead to repetitive strain in your neck. If you wish to compete, most communities have swim programs that allow you to participate in competitive meets. Scuba diving is a good way to break up the monotony of lap swimming. One precaution with scuba diving is to be careful not to arch your low back. Extreme backward bending (or arching) is common among many divers and may lead to back pain. (Swimming is rated a 10.)

Cycling

It is not unusual in Europe and Asia to see people in their 60s and 70s riding a bicycle. Cycling can be a great conditioning exercise, although there is much debate as to whether riding a bicycle is good for your back. Some back experts will say no, because it involves sitting, vibration, forward bending of the low back, and twisting (when a cyclist looks behind while riding). Yet cycling advocates disagree, stating that this is a non-weight bearing sport in which your upper body weight is distributed through the handle bars via your arms and your lower body weight is distributed through the seat, thereby taking pressure off your back. One study of urban bicycle injuries found only 2.6 percent of all cyclist injuries to be located in the low back. The greatest risk to a bicyclist's back occurs when there is a fall. If precautions aren't taken seriously, cycling can be a dangerous sport to your body. Fractures are quite common (especially in the arms), and being struck by a motor vehicle can be life threatening.

If you're an avid on-road or off-road cyclist and this is the only conditioning exercise that you consistently participate in, let me hope that you take every possible precaution. Make sure you wear padded gloves and a bicycle helmet. To reduce twisting, place a mirror on your helmet or bicycle so that you can view the rear (Fig. 8-5). If you ride on the road, use a hybrid or wide tire bike instead of the standard road

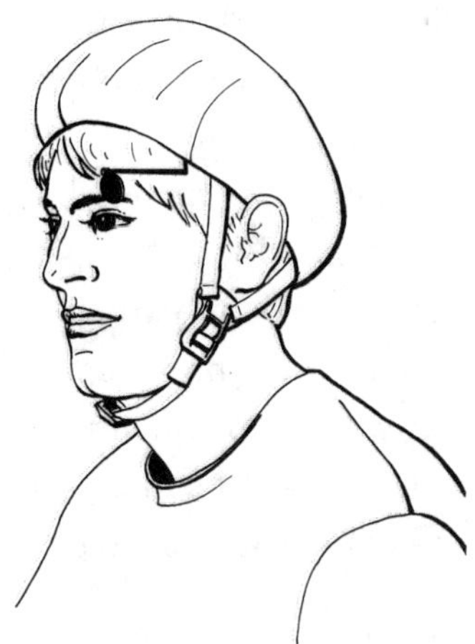

Fig. 8-5. Bicycle helmet and mirror

bike. This will provide a smoother ride with less vibration. Take time to properly adjust your bike to your body frame so that back pain will not develop. In addition, ride on a smooth terrain to minimize the pounding to your body. Above all, ride safely and defensively.

I recommend using a stationary bicycle (Fig. 8-6). Yes, I know there is sitting involved, but if you sit straight and maintain your normal forward curves in your low back and neck, the weight will be distributed down to your pelvis and not on the discs or joints of your back. In addition, this form of exercise can be done at home or at a health club regardless of the weather. (Stationary bike riding is rated a 9.)

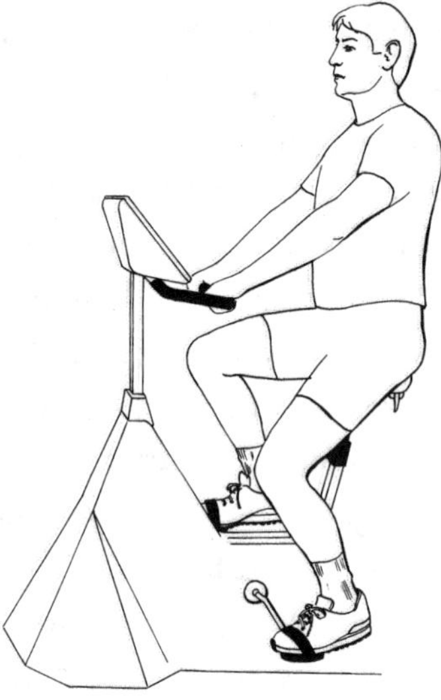

Fig. 8-6. Stationary bike

Rope Skipping

Any boxer will tell you that rope skipping (Fig. 8-7) is an excellent conditioning exercise. Rope skipping shouldn't be done if you are overweight, since it can overload your back. Your bones do, however, need some level of physical loading to help prevent osteoporosis (brittle bones), especially in women. If you prefer to participate in low-impact activities such as swimming or cycling, it is best to alternate your workouts with rope skipping. Always skip on a padded surface to help reduce any chance of injury. (Rope skipping is rated a 9.)

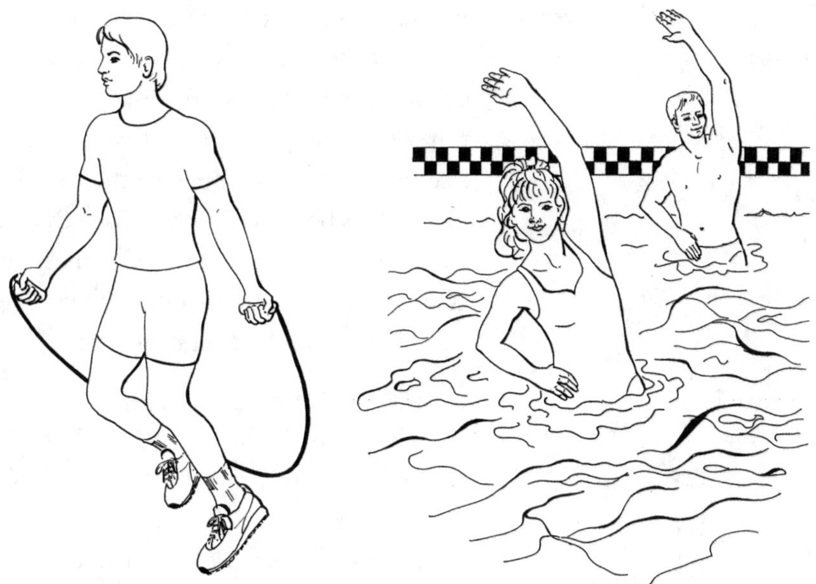

Fig. 8-7. Rope skipping

Fig. 8-8. Water exercise

Water Exercise

Water exercise (Fig. 8-8) has gained in popularity over the past decade for a number of reasons. Water exercise provides a low-impact form of conditioning, which promotes weight loss and may help reduce the risk of injury. In addition, many self-conscious individuals feel comfortable having their bodies hidden under the water. Such people might otherwise be reluctant to participate in a group exercise setting. The unique thing about water exercise is that just about anyone can do it. Having taught an adapted (disabled students) water exercise class for years, I've worked with students who were mentally impaired, blind, arthritic, obese, and paraplegic and who had other physical impairments, including bad backs. All of these people benefited from this form of exercise.

The key to a good water exercise program is finding a good instructor. Unfortunately, water exercise has great variability and no set standards of instruction. Keep in mind that to get the conditioning effect, you need to have continuous body movements against the resistance of the water. Of course, these movements must be back friendly. Vigorous arm and leg movements that don't twist the body or arch the low back are helpful during water exercising. Beware of water exercise programs that move to the beat of music. It is best to move at a pace that is comfortable for your level of fitness to avoid overuse injuries. (Water exercise with proper instruction is rated a 9.)

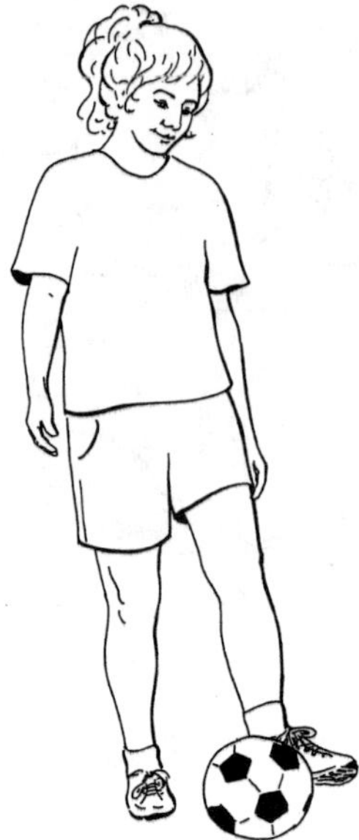

Fig. 8-9. Soccer

Soccer and Basketball

Although soccer and basketball players can experience back pain, these sports haven't been found to put one's back at risk. Therefore, if you enjoy participating in team sports, soccer (Fig. 8-9) or basketball (Fig. 8-10) might be for you. For these sports to be considered a conditioning exercise, there must be a continuous rate of activity. This can be difficult with time-outs and sharing playing time with others on the team. However, if done at a continuous level, these sports will give you quite a workout, unless, of course, you're a goalkeeper.

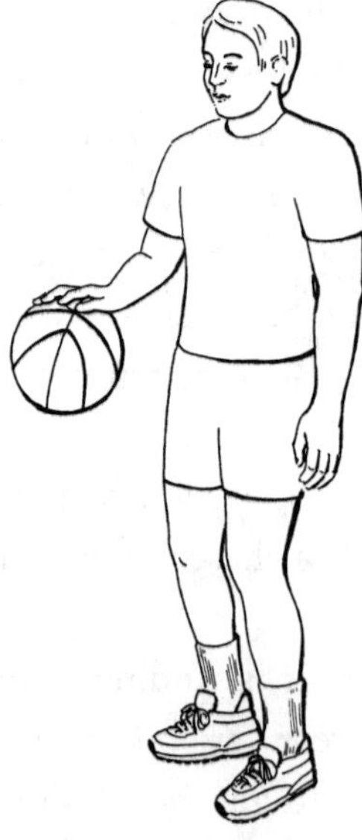

Fig. 8-10. Basketball

Although soccer and basketball are designed as noncontact sports, they can be very physical. Since ankle and knee injuries are common, it is best to avoid as much body contact as possible to help reduce risk of injury. For example, if you love to play basketball but dislike body contact and you like to play guard or forward, this game is for you. However, if you prefer playing center and love to work the boards, you might want to consider another conditioning exercise. If you like to play soccer, avoid using your head to hit the ball when possible. This may help prevent wear and tear to your neck. It is important when you play soccer to give more consideration when stretching the back of your thigh, hip flexor, and inner thigh muscles. These muscles have typically been found to be tight among soccer players and, if left unchecked, can lead to back pain. For the competitive individual, most communities have recreational leagues. If you alternate between soccer and basketball, you could play competitive sports practically all year long. (Because of the risk of injury from body contact, soccer and basketball are rated an 8.)

Dancing

Dancing (Fig. 8-11) is a great way to have fun and still get a workout, although not all dance routines are safe. For example, the twist, as the name implies, twists the back in vigorous movements and should be avoided. Because there are so many different types of dances (especially cultural dances), may I suggest that it would be best to eliminate any movements from your favorite dance routine that aren't back friendly, such as twisting, forward bending, extreme backward bending, and lifting, catching, or supporting your partner. Some dance routines, such as tap, ballroom, or slow dancing, can be easily modified by avoiding these undesirable movements. Dance instructors can be helpful in advising you how to modify your movements. In addition, you might need an instructor to fit alternative movements into the normal rhythm of your specific dance routine. Remember,

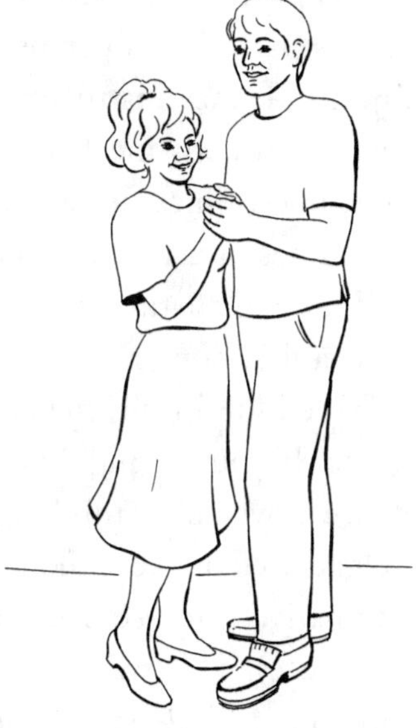

Fig. 8-11. Dancing

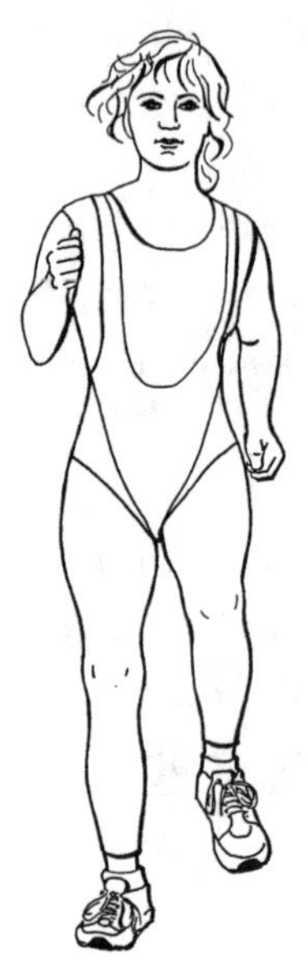

Fig. 8-12. Aerobic dance

for dancing to be considered a conditioning workout, it must be done on a continuous level. (Tap dancing is rated a 10.)

Probably the most popular dance routine used strictly for exercise is aerobic dancing (Fig. 8-12). Like water exercise, the quality of this form of exercise is determined in large part by the dance instructor. With that in mind, the Aerobics and Fitness Association of America (AFAA) has determined certain safety standards that are recommended and taught for aerobic dance instructors. Certification of these guidelines has become mandatory by many health clubs and colleges in the hiring of aerobic dance instructors.

The risks associated with aerobic dancing are mainly from overuse and improper use of body mechanics, which can lead to injuries. Dance instructors should use low-impact movements with the proper body mechanics mentioned in this book or in the AFAA guidelines. Since not all certified AFAA instructors use the AFAA guidelines, it is best to shop around until you find an instructor who will adhere to the movements. In addition to using proper body mechanics, don't forget to wear a good pair of aerobic dance shoes designed specifically to help reduce the impact upon your muscles and joints. If you are highly conditioned, be sure not to overexaggerate dance movements, thinking it will help you to become more fit. Often exaggerated or overzealous movements can lead to back pain. A good alternative is to use hand weights between 1/2 pound and 2 pounds (no more). This will add resistance while maintaining normal body movements. If 2-pound hand weights aren't enough to maintain your fitness level, move on to a different conditioning exercise. (Aerobic dancing done with proper instruction is rated an 8.)

ACTIVITIES TO AVOID

Any sport or activity that has a tendency to use one side of the body repetitively should be avoided or, at the very least, minimized. Such recreational activities include golf, fencing, bowling, the overhead serving stroke of tennis, batting and throwing in baseball or softball, even serving and spiking in volleyball. The one-sided motions of these activities lead to muscle imbalances, which create more wear and tear to the joints in your back. When you combine twisting to a one-sided sport, such as golfing, you're placing more stress upon your discs and joints, thereby compounding the risk of developing back pain.

Beware of fitness gurus who preach that you should work as many muscles as possible during your conditioning routine. It is true that you will burn more calories with more muscle activity, although it is more important to work your heart at its proper level and to perform certain movements while avoiding others. This will prevent you from putting your heart and back at risk, which is more important than burning a few more calories. Beware of such fitness devices as stationary bikes, treadmills, rowing machines, and cross-country skiing machines that use arm movements in front of your body, since these arm movements place your mid-back and your neck at further risk.

CHAPTER 9

Conditioning Guidelines

NOW THAT YOU'VE LEARNED the types of conditioning exercises that are recommended, let's address some misconceptions regarding the training effect of these activities. Many individuals believe that if they walk on and off during the day, they must be in good condition. An opposite myth, held by many, relates to the saying "no pain, no gain," where individuals don't feel they are getting conditioned unless they push themselves to the limit during every workout.

How do you know, then, whether you are getting the proper training for your heart, lungs, and overall body? The American College of Sports Medicine has recommended certain guidelines for conditioning activities that will help you to exercise at a healthy rate. The quality and amount of training depend on the frequency, duration, and intensity of the conditioning activity as well as the level of fitness of the individual. The highly conditioned adult will be able to exercise at a higher intensity, for longer duration and more frequently than an unfit adult who hasn't exercised in years. To fully comprehend this concept, let's discuss each guideline in detail.

Frequency: This literally means the number of times per week that you exercise. Maintaining your conditioning level requires at least two to three workouts per week. Frequency depends of course upon the duration and intensity of each workout and your level of fitness.

Duration: This means the amount of time spent exercising during a workout. An unfit individual may be able to exercise for only minutes at a time before the conditioning exercise becomes too intense, while a triathlete might last ten hours.

Intensity: This basically means how hard you work out. High-intensity workouts pose a greater risk of orthopedic injuries and put your heart at risk. Of course, performing exercises without a certain duration and without some intensity does not qualify as a conditioning exercise, since your body isn't being worked hard enough.

When you combine frequency, duration, and intensity, you can vary the level of a workout to match your capability. Knowing how to change the intensity of your conditioning exercise is important because your level of fitness can vary drastically throughout your life, even from year to year.

In addition, certain conditioning exercises are more intense than others when performed at the same duration and frequency. Cycling at a pace of 15 mph is more intense than walking. To get the same workout effect of cycling at 15 mph, you'll need to increase your time spent walking. In other words, low-intensity conditioning workouts can be similar in training effect to high-intensity workouts if you're willing to spend more time exercising. This added time may be well spent when you keep in mind that high-intensity conditioning exercises increase your risk of orthopedic and cardiovascular (heart, blood vessel, and lung) injuries. People also tend to stay with an exercise program when it is done at a low rather than a high intensity level.

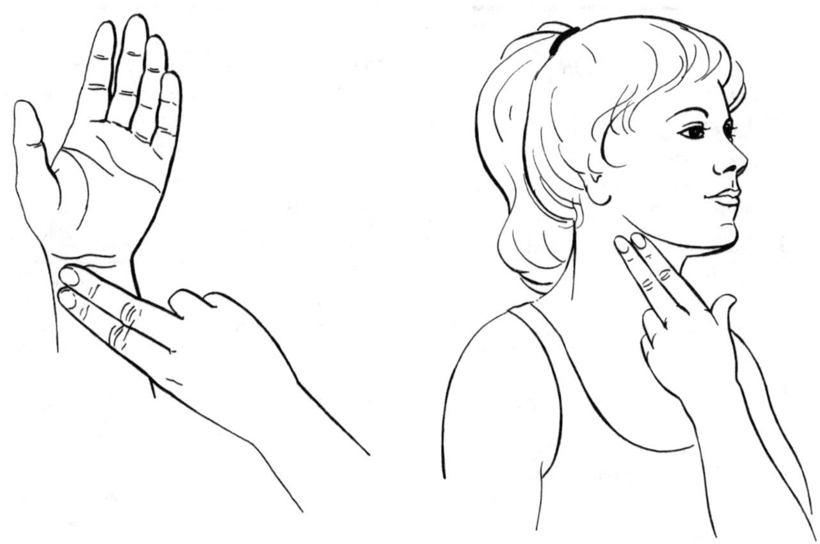

Fig. 9-1. Wrist pulse

Fig. 9-2. Neck pulse

HOW TO DETERMINE YOUR INTENSITY LEVEL

To find the right pace for you during conditioning, try using a wireless heart rate monitor or learn how to find your target heart rate (THR). By monitoring your heart rate, you'll be able to determine whether you are over or under training.

To find your resting heart rate or pulse, slightly touch the thumb side of your wrist or the area next to your Adam's apple with your first two fingers (Fig. 9-1, 9-2). Count the beats for 10 seconds, then multiply by 6, which will give you your resting heart rate. To get an accurate resting heart rate, check your pulse when you first wake up in the morning. Once you are able to find your resting heart rate, you're ready to find your individualized target heart rate. Table 9-1 shows the formula for calculating the THR of a 35-year-old. (Fill in the blank formula with your age and resting heart rate.)

TABLE 9-1

FORMULA FOR CALCULATING THR

Start here	220	220
Subtract your age	- 35	- ___
Maximum heart rate	185	
Subtract your resting heart rate	- 72	- ___
	113	
Choose your percentage of maximum heart rate* (for this example, we'll use 55%).		
	x.55	x
	62	
Add your resting heart rate	+ 72	+
Your THR	134	
Divide by 6	÷ 6	÷ 6
Your 10-second THR	= 22	=

*Beginning exercisers and those who wish to burn fat should exercise at a low-intensity level, which is 50%-65% of maximum heart rate. Those whose intention is just to maintain a current level of fitness and body composition should exercise at a moderate pace, which is 65%-75% of maximum heart rate. Those capable of working out at a competitive fitness level may wish to have a high intensity workout, which is 75%-80% of maximum heart rate.

The formula in Table 9-1 indicates that the 35-year- old individual with a resting heart rate of 72 will have a target heart rate of 134. If this person is a beginning exerciser, his or her 10-second THR range is between 22 and 24. This same person who is maintaining a physically fit level would have a 10-second THR range between 24 and 26. The same individual who is fit enough to compete would have a 10-second THR range between 26 and 27.

In addition to using your target heart rate for determining your intensity, you can use the Borg Scale (Table 9-2). Gunnar Borg, a Swedish psychologist, found that people are accurately able to feel different levels of intensity as they work out. The more you exercise, the better you will be able to judge the different levels of intensity. This scale should be used in conjunction with your target heart rate. This way you will have two reliable methods to determine your intensity level.

TABLE 9-2

BORG'S PERCEIVED EXERTION SCALE

6. No exertion at all
7. Extremely light
8.
9. Very light
10.
11. Light
12.
13. Somewhat hard
14.
15. Hard
16.
17. Very hard
18.
19. Extremely hard
20. Maximal exertion

The Borg sale is an approximation of your target heart rate. If you multiply your perceived level of exertion by 10, the number should closely match your target heart rate. The 35-year-old in our example with a resting heart rate of 72 would match the scale if he or she felt that the workout was "somewhat hard." (Since 13 x 10 = 130, this is close to 134, which is this individual's target heart rate.) It is recommended that a rating between 12 and 14 on the Borg Sale be used for a health-related conditioning workout, since this gives you a low-to moderate-intensity level.

Generally, you can determine your workout level by your breathing during your workout. If your breathing is so hard that you can't talk during your workout, you're exercising too hard. If you can talk yet feel you're a little out of breath, your level is somewhat hard. If you can talk without any change in breathing, your workout can be classified as light.

GETTING IN SHAPE

When starting a conditioning program, each individual will have different fitness and health status, age, and goals. For example, a person in his or her early twenties who hasn't exercised in a year will progress faster to a higher fitness level than a middle-aged adult who has never maintained an exercise routine. In fact, the severely unfit individual or the person recovering from a heart attack will have to exercise at such a low intensity that it may take 6 to 12 months before being able to exercise at a level that will maintain even a minimal level of fitness.

Since it may be dangerous to increase your conditioning level too rapidly, the American College of Sports Medicine has developed three stages of progression: initial, improvement, maintenance. These stages should be used anytime you wish to increase your fitness level. If you are currently engaged in a regular conditioning program yet wish to increase your fitness level, simply move on to the improvement stage of progression.

The majority of participants will need to start in the initial conditioning stage. The U.S. Preventive Services Task Force has estimated that at least 40 percent of our population is physically inactive and another 40 percent exercises at levels below those recommended to achieve health-related benefits. It is always best to start your initial conditioning stage at a lower intensity than you calculated for your target heart rate as a beginning exerciser. When determining your intensity, choose 40 percent to 60 percent of your maximum heart rate. If you haven't been fit for years, choose the 40 percent intensity level and slowly build up your fitness level. Modifications will be made in the intensity, duration, and frequency of your workouts, depending on your initial level of fitness and how you feel during and after your conditioning workout. Eventually, duration should last at least 10 to 15 minutes two to three times a week. If you go above your THR early or feel poorly after using this time frame, lower your intensity so that you will be able to work out for at least 10 to 15 minutes.

Keep in mind that the initial stage was designed to use low-intensity conditioning to avoid any soreness or discomfort associated with starting an exercise program. Progress will be slow. The key to this stage is to make it easy for you to adapt and to get you prepared physically and mentally for a routine conditioning program. So make it easy and fun. This stage typically lasts four to six weeks, although people with heart disease might be instructed by their doctor to work for ten weeks in the initial stage.

As suggested by its name, the improvement stage has the participant rapidly progress in his or her conditioning level. Begin this stage within your target heart rate. Remember that if you're a beginning exerciser, your percentage of maximum heart rate is between 50 percent and 65 percent. If you are already fit and wish to increase your level of fitness, your percentage of maximum heart rate is between 65 percent and 85 percent.

It is up to you to modify your intensity, duration, and frequency to a level that will feel "somewhat hard" and match your target heart rate. During this stage, you're putting your body under considerable physical stress. Without some physical stress, you won't improve, yet too much stress can be detrimental to your health. Therefore, periodically check your pulse rate during your workout to make sure you are at the appropriate level. Don't forget to listen to your body. There will be days when you simply won't feel as strong. When this happens, just slow down to the point where you feel comfortable. The more you exercise, the better you will become at judging your appropriate intensity by how you are feeling.

Approximately every two to three weeks, increase your duration of exercise. Eventually, you will want to exercise for at least 20 to 30 minutes. The frequency should be built up to three times a week. If you're fit enough to be at a competitive level, five times a week may be appropriate. Before increasing intensity at this level, you should already be exercising 20 to 30 minutes three times a week. Once you increase intensity, lower your duration and slowly build back up to the duration you desire.

You will want sooner or later to enter into the maintenance conditioning stage. Most individuals will end the improvement stage when they meet the minimum level of conditioning and not when they have reached a competitive fitness level. This is perfectly all right, since you will get the health-related benefits of exercise that you are seeking with the minimum level of conditioning. This allows you more time to live your life and meet your busy schedule while maintaining a fit back and body.

To maintain your conditioning level, you must participate in an exercise program that has a duration of 20 to 30 minutes at your THR, is performed at a frequency of three times a week, and gives you a target heart rate where your intensity is calculated at 65 percent to 85 percent of your maximum heart rate. Your level of fitness will determine what intensity rate you wish to work at. For example, a person may need a THR calculated at 65 percent of maximum for a 30-minute workout just to maintain his or her level of fitness, while another person in slightly better shape may need a THR calculated at 75 percent maximum for a 30-minute workout to maintain his or her level of fitness. In addition, you will need to monitor your breathing rate during exercise to make sure you stay within the "somewhat hard" level of conditioning. Therefore, as you can see, maintaining your conditioning level doesn't have to be grueling or time consuming. In fact, the minimum amount of time is only one hour per week.

As a physical education instructor, I have occasionally met students who believe that since they are "in shape" they don't need to exercise regularly. Some of these students may be conditioned enough to swim 700 yards in 12 minutes, which means they would rate "good" in a fitness test. The point that I wish to make is that if you don't maintain a regular exercise program, you will eventually get out of shape. Also, for your body to have health-related benefits (strong heart, lungs, bones, and back) from exercise, you will need to exercise regularly. It is the process and not necessarily the product of exercise that gives us health benefits.

OVEREXERCISING

Individuals with certain personality behaviors tend to overwork or overtrain. People who are impatient, achievement oriented, or highly competitive tend to push themselves beyond their THR and comfort zone when conditioning. Excessive exercisers have even been known to work out despite pain and injury. If you happen to fall into this category, remember that the philosophy of "the more, the better" as it applies to conditioning is dangerous and should be avoided. Usually individuals overexercise themselves by improperly combining the intensity, duration, and frequency of their workout. In addition, they may be misinterpreting the "somewhat hard" feeling with "hard" or "very hard," thereby overworking themselves. Even the most experienced exerciser has at times pushed him or herself too hard. It is therefore important to learn some signs and symptoms of overexertion. If any of the first four symptoms in the following list occur, seek immediate care from your doctor.

1. Pain/injury
2. Tightness in chest
3. Dizziness
4. Increased frequency in colds
5. Headache
6. Constant tiredness
7. Sleeplessness
8. Soreness

Always remember that since your are exercising to improve your health and not to create health problems, you should avoid overexertion from exercise. If you are training to compete or have a tendency to overtrain, a good way to monitor yourself to prevent overexertion is by checking your pulse rate and body weight daily.

For years, many endurance coaches recommended that athletes take their resting heart rate for one minute upon arising in the morning. If the athletes had a ten percent increase in their resting heart rate, the coach would taper off their subsequent workouts. Recently, this procedure was changed to make it more sensitive to overexertion. It is now recommended that upon awakening and while still lying down, you should take your pulse for 15 seconds. You should then stand and immediately take it again. There normally is a difference of three to five beats. If you trained too hard the previous day, thc difference may be five to eight beats. If this happens, it is recommended that you work out at an easier pace until you wake up with your normal heart rate.

You can lose a lot of water by perspiring during a strong workout. A hot and humid day could have an additional effect upon your body through water loss during a workout. Without proper amounts of water within your body, you can develop cramps, heat exhaustion, or possibly heat stroke. A good way to monitor your water level is by body weight. Your weight should be checked just before and immediately after exercise and again the following morning.

According to the American Dietetic Association, if you haven't returned to within one to two pounds of your normal weight by the following morning, subsequent workouts should be temporarily tapered off until your normal weight is regained. The ADA recommends that you drink 16 ounces of fluid for each pound lost before your next workout.

CHAPTER 10

Weight Training

MOST BACK PAIN IS DIAGNOSED to be the result of a strain or sprain of the muscles or ligaments of the spine. Repeated strain/sprain injuries lead to more wear and tear of the joints and discs in your back, thus causing severe and sometimes permanent damage. When you break a bone, it heals stronger. If you tear a muscle or ligament (strain/sprain), however, it heals with weaker and less elastic tissue, thereby making you more susceptible to further muscle and ligament injuries.

HEALTH BENEFITS OF WEIGHT TRAINING

You've been told to sit and stand with good posture or to lift objects using your legs and not your back because doing so lessens the chance of your developing a strain/sprain injury. Another excellent way to help prevent back strain/sprain injuries is to increase your muscle strength and muscle endurance so that you can increase the amount of physical loading upon your muscles and ligaments, again reducing your chance of developing a strain/sprain.

The best way to increase your strength is through weight training. To the surprise of many, weight training is no longer viewed as a form of self-torture used solely among our youth to achieve what some consider to be attractiveness. Recent evidence suggests that weight training may help to increase strength even among the elderly. Does this mean you need to become a bodybuilder and spend hours a day pumping iron in your local gym? Of course not! But it does mean that you can no longer afford to overlook this form of exercise. The health-related benefits of weight training are a must not only for a healthy back but also for a healthy body.

It can't be emphasized enough that a fit back is dependent upon a fit body. Your back is connected and supported by your upper and lower limbs. To prevent strain/sprain in your back, you need to develop strength throughout your body. This may seem obvious, but many individuals, including fitness experts and some health care providers, have mistakenly concentrated on exercises directly related to the back without considering the total body. You can work the entire body through weight training.

As a person ages, he or she will lose muscle tissue, and with most individuals, the existing muscle tissue will shrink from inactivity. Such changes in aging muscles will create two profound effects: they cause muscle weakness, and they lower our body metabolism (the rate at which we burn calories). As stated earlier, muscle weakness can contribute to the likelihood of developing back strain/sprain injuries. In addition, since strong muscles help to create strong bones, muscle weakness may increase the risk for developing osteoporosis. Also, being inactive for a prolonged period will create more muscle weakness, causing slow movements and probably making you more dependent upon others to perform your daily activities as you get older.

Muscle weakness in the elderly can result in individuals becoming frail. Studies have shown that extreme muscle weakness in the elderly can lead to more falls, a major threat to an older person's health. Falls are a leading cause of injury, disability, and even death among the elderly. Fortunately, weight training has been found to help curb many of these conditions commonly associated with aging. Lifting weights can increase the size of your muscle mass, help to strengthen your bones, and give you more strength and muscle endurance, even in your later years.

Another effect of increased activity is a decrease in body fat. Since the muscles in one's body burn calories, muscles that have shrunk from inactivity will hinder one's ability to maintain a normal body weight. As a result, weight training is needed to enlarge your muscles, which will help counteract any muscle loss as you age and improve your muscles' ability to burn calories. Bigger muscles worked during conditioning will burn more calories and help to increase your metabolism while resting.

SAFETY FACTORS

Since weight training doesn't get your heart pumping as hard as conditioning exercises do, weight training alone won't burn body fat. This also means that you don't need to breathe heavily when lifting to have enough energy to perform your exercises. Since these exercises require short and quick movements, you already have enough energy present in your body to execute these movements. Although breathing isn't necessary to produce sufficient energy when performing certain exercises, it should be emphasized that proper breathing plays a major role in safe weight training.

Most fitness experts believe that it is best to exhale when lifting and inhale in the recovery phase. Holding your breath during weight training increases blood pressure and decreases bloodflow to the brain which may cause fainting. Some fitness experts believe that holding your breath or breathing out at the last moment during lifting provides more stability to your spine. Since injuries to a back usually create instability, this may be a good procedure if you aren't suffering from high blood pressure or a heart condition. If you have injured your back and wish to begin to lift weights, consult with your doctor before beginning and ask which breathing technique is better for you.

Proper clothing is required when weight lifting. Loose-fitting clothes are essential to allow unrestricted movements while lifting.

Shoes with an elevated heel create a physical stress to your back and should be avoided. Be aware that some athletic (i.e., running) shoes have an elevated heel. A flat and wide base athletic shoe will provide more stability when lifting weights and are recommended. If you wish to prevent callouses on your hands while lifting weights, you may want to wear weight-training gloves.

As a preventive measure, many people wear a lifting belt when working out to help support their back. In fact, research suggests that the use of a belt when lifting helps to increase pressure in the abdominal region. This may help reduce compressive forces placed upon your discs in the back, thereby improving lifting safety. Unfortunately, if you wear the belt constantly when lifting, your deep stomach muscles will weaken, thus increasing your risk of injury if you happen to lift without your belt. As a result, it is recommended you wear a belt only when you're lifting near your maximum and only during certain lifts (squats, pulling exercises, and leg lunges).

Probably the most important injury prevention measure during weight lifting is to lift using correct techniques. Pay special attention to the instructions in the "How to Perform Exercise" feature with most of the exercises in this chapter. You may save yourself from an injury. In addition, have the staff at your health club demonstrate the use of the equipment and proper lifting technique for each exercise. The more information you receive on the use of equipment and lifting techniques, the better your workout and the less likelihood of your injuring yourself.

Certain types of weight-training equipment are safer than others. While there isn't one manufacturer of equipment that is completely back-friendly, I recommend that you use weight machines for most of your lifts. Since this type of equipment doesn't need to be loaded, you have less risk of dropping the weight on yourself than you do with free weights (barbell, dumbbells). Having a workout partner while lifting weights is still recommended to make sure your lifting mechanics are proper and that you lift the weight smoothly and not with jerky or rapid motions, which place unneeded stress upon your back.

BEFORE YOU BEGIN

Your routine will consist of sets, repetitions, and amount lifted during most exercises. For example, you could do arm curls for three sets, 10 repetitions each set, at the weight of 40 pounds. In other words, you lift a 40-pound weight ten times (repetitions), which makes one set, which you'll repeat three times. At this point, you've finished the exercise of arm curls.

Performing two to three sets of eight to twelve repetitions at a moderate intensity two times a week for each weight-training exercise is recommended. Such a routine will be sufficient to maintain and even increase your muscle strength, muscle endurance, and size. To give your body proper rest, it is best to alternate body parts when weight training. On a four times a week workout, it is best to work the upper body one day and the lower body during the next workout. This way you work your upper and lower body two times a week. This routine is recommended because if you do miss one workout, you will still maintain your muscle strength and endurance level. Keep in mind that the effects of weight training are short-lived. To maintain your current muscle strength and muscle endurance, you need to weight train each muscle group at least once a week or you will lose the benefits.

Table 10-1 shows a suggested back-friendly routine for a four times a week weight-training workout.

TABLE 10-1
BACK-FRIENDLY ROUTINE

Monday and Thursday	Tuesday and Friday
Upper Body	Lower Body
Standing shoulder shrugs	Back extensions
Pull-downs	Knee extensors
Neck exercises	Lunges
Push-downs	Toe raises
Overhead press	Leg push
Incline bench press	Leg pulls
Bench press	Hanging knee raises
Curls	Leg curls

It is important to work the common underdeveloped muscle groups related to proper posture at the beginning of your workout. Because these muscles should be worked first while you're fresh and before you become tired, I recommend that the upper and lower body be worked in the exact order as listed in Table 10-1 to achieve maximum benefit. (Feel free to alternate days of the week in which you work out to best fit your personal schedule.)

Whether lifting two or three sets per workout, you need to increase your weight when the twelfth repetition on the last set becomes easy. Increase your weight by ten pounds at a time. Then start lifting each set at eight repetitions instead of twelve. As your strength increases and the lifting becomes easier, increase your repetitions from eight to ten to twelve. Only when you're able to do twelve repetitions easily on the last set are you ready to again increase your weight.

Besides the two to three sets of lifting that you need to do during your strengthening routine, it is important that you do an additional lighter set before each exercise. This warm-up set will help prepare certain muscles, tendons, and ligaments for your total workout. Your shoulders and knees are at most risk for an injury during weight training. To prevent injuries from occurring, a warm-up set is needed prior to every weight-training exercise. Therefore, you will have a specific warm-up aside from the general body (stretching) warm-up before lifting. You should do your weight-lifting warm-up set at 50 percent to 60 percent of your normal lifting weight. For example, if you lift 300 pounds on your toe-raising exercise, the weight for your warm-up set should be approximately 150 pounds. It is best to do your warm-ups for eight to ten repetitions.

ABDOMINAL EXERCISES

You also need to work your abdominal muscles before you lift weights. After your full-body warm-up and before working your upper or lower body, do the following four exercises to help strengthen your abdominal region. Because strong abdominal muscles are essential to maintaining a healthy back, I recommend that they be worked at least four times a week.

Working the abdominal muscles is frequently done incorrectly, if done at all. It is no wonder that most people have weak abdominal muscles. Before discussing how to exercise these muscles, let's discuss some common misconceptions. When most people think of working their abdominal muscles, they think of sit-ups. Many people are further mistaken into thinking that sit-ups will get rid of the fat surrounding their stomach. Not only do sit-ups poorly work the abdominal muscles, but they don't burn fat around the stomach.

Beware of anyone who tries to sell you an exercise device that tones your muscles in your abdomen or thighs and implies that you will lose fat. THESE EXERCISE DEVICES ALONE WILL NOT BURN FAT. If you wish to have a flat stomach or firm thighs, you'll need to participate regularly in a complete exercise program and eat properly. Even then, you'll lose fat throughout your body and not in one specific spot.

Another misconception deals with straight-leg sit-ups, which can actually cause posture and back problems. Two thirds of the straight leg sit-ups are the work of the hip flexor muscles. If these muscles become overdeveloped, you might develop an increased forward curve in the low back (swayback), which increases the stress applied to the low back, thereby possibly creating an injury.

Abdominal exercises shouldn't be done on a weight machine. These popular machines involve the hip flexor muscles to an undesirable level and require improper body movements. The following floor exercises will work best to isolate your abdominals. When working these muscles, make sure not to arch your back and keep your knees bent when advised to do so. It is recommended to build up to at least 50 repetitions for each abdominal exercise. Start with the tougher exercises while you're fresh and able to concentrate on the proper technique.

SIDE SIT-UPS

This exercise is done to strengthen the abdominal muscles and the muscles on one side of your lower back. This is a difficult exercise for the average person to perform. Don't get frustrated if you cannot start this exercise with 50 repetitions. If you can do only one repetition, simply do more sets to build your strength.

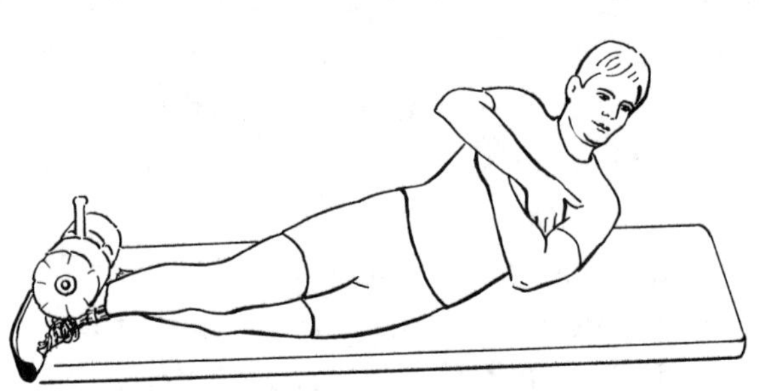

Fig. 10-1. Side sit-ups

Always do this exercise on a padded surface. While lying on your side, lift your upper body from the bench or mat with your arms folded across your chest. If you don't have a workout partner to hold your feet, hook your feet under a sit-up bench. Then repeat with the other side. This will develop your oblique stomach muscles.

Do not jerk your body up. It is important to keep your body straight and not to twist it. Make sure not to push off with your elbow (Fig. 10-1).

REVERSE CRUNCHES

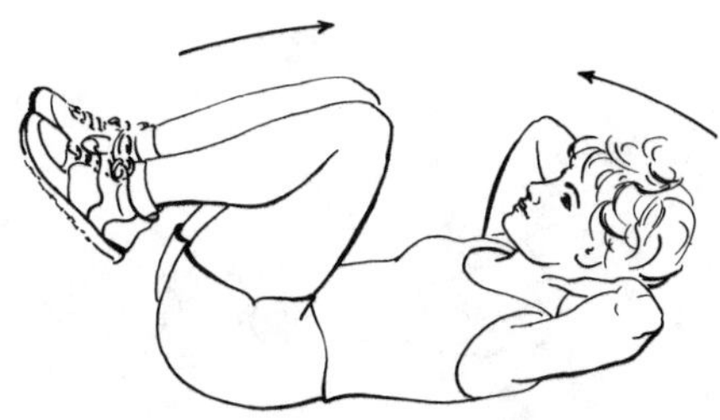

Fig. 10-2. Reverse crunches

Lie flat on your back with your legs elevated until your knees are directly above your hip joints. With your hands behind your head, slowly raise your upper body and knees toward each other. Pull your knees toward your chest while lifting your shoulders off the floor about 10 degrees. Upon lowering the legs, make sure to stop when your knees are again directly above your hips. Be careful to keep your neck straight. Do not curl your head forward. Place minimal pressure on your head from your hands and lift your body straight upward about 10 degrees (Fig. 10-2). This works both your lower and upper abdominal area.

CRUNCHES

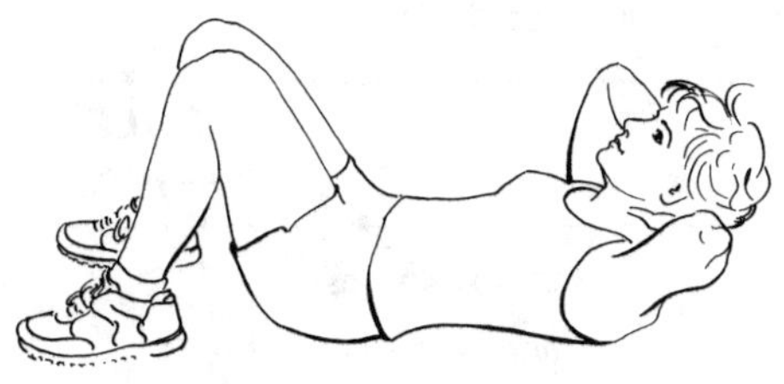

Fig. 10-3. Crunches

Lie on your back in the standard bent-knee sit-up position. Slowly raise your shoulders and upper back off the floor. Lift your shoulders off the floor about 10 degrees and hold for a second before returning to starting position. Be careful to keep your neck straight. Do not pull your hands against the back of your head. To make sure you don't bend your neck, keep your eyes focused on the ceiling and not toward your knees. One repetition consists of lifting and lowering your upper back and shoulders (Fig. 10-3).

1/4 SIT-UPS

Lie flat on your back with your legs elevated until your knees are directly above your hip joints. Cross your feet and place your hands behind your head. Lift and lower your head, shoulders, and upper back

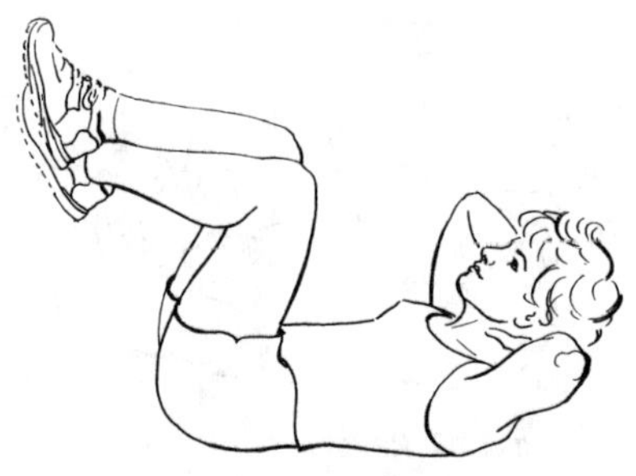

Fig. 10-4. 1/4 sit-ups

as quickly as possible. Keep your neck straight with minimal pressure on your head from your hands. Lift your body straight up and not toward the knees (Fig. 10-4). This exercise mainly works your upper abdominal area.

WEIGHT-TRAINING WORKOUT

If you prefer a two-day workout or select it simply because it fits your schedule better, follow the routine in Table 10-2. This routine will have you working your upper and lower body on the same day. This order of exercises for the two-day routine (1-16) was chosen specifically for its importance in maintaining a healthy back. The remainder of this section describes how to do the exercises listed in Tables 10-1 and 10-2.

TABLE 10-2
TWO-DAY WEIGHT TRAINING ROUTINE

1. Back extensions	9. Leg pulls
2. Standing shoulder shrugs	10. Toe raises
3. Pull-downs	11. Leg curls
4. Neck exercises	12. Overhead press
5. Hanging knee raises	13. Push-downs
6. Knee extensors	14. Curls
7. Lunges	15. Bench press
8. Leg push	16. Incline bench press

BACK EXERCISES

Low Back

Of all the weight-training exercises found in the back-friendly workout, low-back exercises are the most controversial. You probably wouldn't think so, yet many experts find it difficult to agree on which low-back exercises to recommend. For example, in the standing position, loading your back with weight and bending forward poses a severe risk to the discs of your spine. Yet many fitness instructors and physical educators recommend this type of exercise as a way to strengthen the muscles of your back.

Your low-back muscles are used to lift your body upward from a forward bending position and to maintain your upright posture. Yet when you bend forward, it is the low back that supports the weight of your upper body. When you place weights on your shoulders and bend forward (Fig. 10-5), you have not only more compression of your discs but also more loading upon your ligaments and joints of your back, causing more wear and tear.

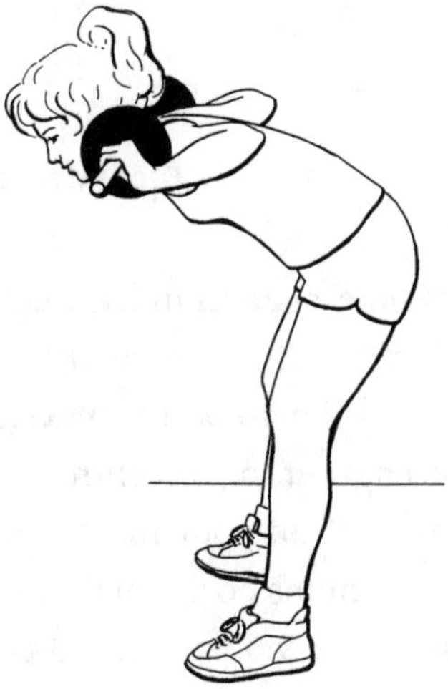

Fig. 10-5. Back exercise to avoid

You can strengthen your muscles without overloading your discs. If you hang upside down, you decompress (unload) your discs. As a result, inversion and back extension machines were developed so that your legs and waist are horizontal while your upper body is vertical. From this position, you lift your upper body until your whole body is horizontal. Your back muscles will strengthen by lifting your upper body weight. In addition, while you're hanging upside down, your body weight is distributed onto the machine and not on your low back.

It is best to use an inversion back-strengthening machine. These machines have you bend your knees, placing less stress on the back of your thighs. Back extension machines will have you keep one or both legs straight (Fig 10-6). This will strengthen the back thigh muscles, which if overdeveloped can lead to back pain.

Never use inversion machines to work your abdominal muscles, since curling your body forward while upside down will create extreme

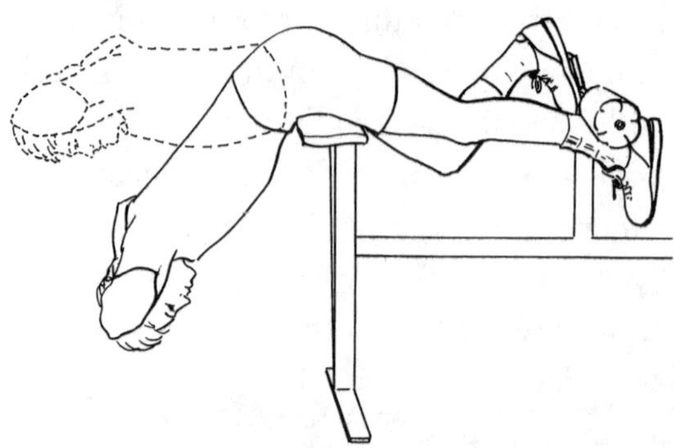

Fig. 10-6. Back extension machine

forward bending. In addition, never twist while hanging upside down. Being inverted stretches your spine. Twisting done while your discs and joints are stretched is a risky movement and should be avoided.

For the young or middle-aged fit individual with no prior back injury and for those who do this exercise regularly, this exercise is recommended (Fig. 10-7).

How to perform exercise: There are a number of inversion back-strengthening machines. Ask your fitness instructor how to place yourself on your machine. Once you are hanging upside down with your thighs horizontal, slowly lift your back up to the point where your spine is level with your thighs (Fig. 10-6). Never lift your upper body above the horizontal position, since doing so will arch your low back.

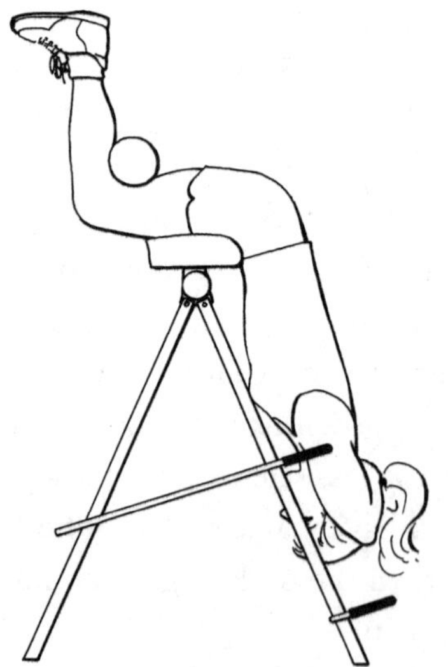

Fig. 10-7a. Inversion machine

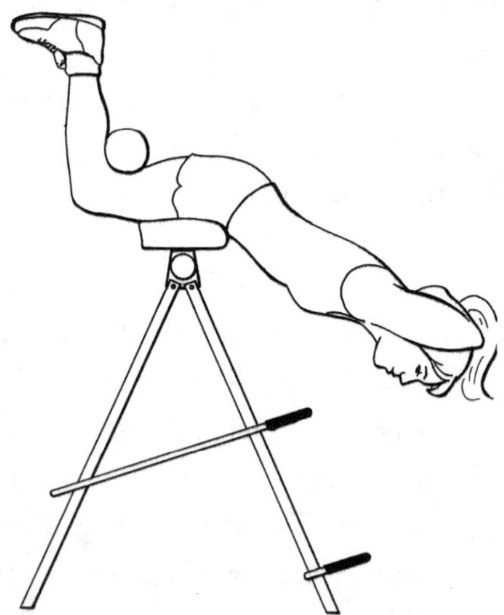

Fig. 10-7b. Inversion machine

Depending on your age and fitness level, you may need to do a different low-back exercise. For the unfit, middle-aged, or elderly, it is best to perform this exercise with no weights and with minimal forward or backward bending. This exercise can be accomplished in the following manner.

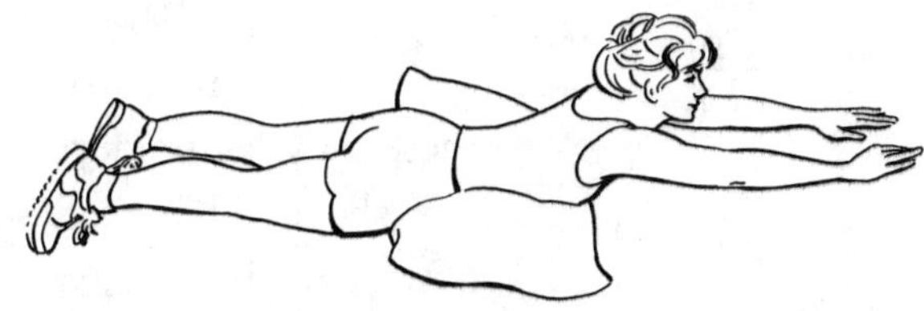

Fig. 10-8. Back extensions

How to perform exercise: Lying face down on a pillow located between your hips and your chest, raise your arms, head, and back slightly (a few degrees) upward (do not arch your low back) and hold to the count of 10 (Fig. 10-8). Repeat until you have done three sets.

Upper and Mid-Back

The upper and middle back muscles help you to maintain good posture by pulling your shoulders back. If these muscles aren't developed adequately, you may develop rounded shoulders (Fig. 10-9).

STANDING SHOULDER SHRUGS

You can do this exercise with dumbbells, with a barbell, or on a machine. This exercise works the upper back.

How to perform exercise: Hold the weights shoulder width with your arms straight. Lift your shoulders toward your ears, then lower them while keeping your arms straight (Fig. 10-10).

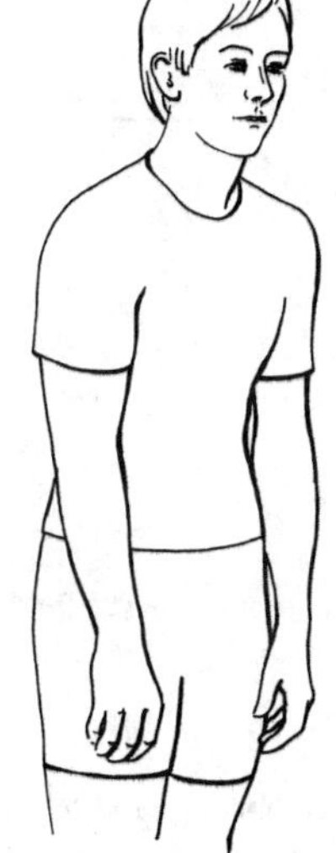

Fig. 10-9. Rounded shoulder posture

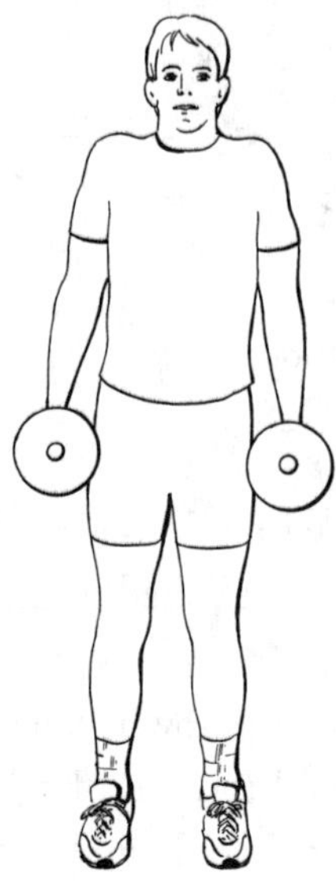

Fig. 10-10. Shoulder shrugs

PULL-DOWNS

This exercise works the mid-back. When these muscles are developed, it gives the back a V-shape. This exercise is done on a pull-down machine.

How to perform exercise: From a standing position, grab the bar of the pull-down machine, then sit or kneel. Some pull-down machines are high enough for you to stand at. I recommend standing during this exercise rather than sitting or kneeling, if possible. Using a wide grip, pull the bar down behind your neck while facing forward. Pull your arms and shoulders back far enough so that you don't tilt your head forward (which strains your neck) and so that you don't hit your head or your neck with the bar (Fig. 10-11).

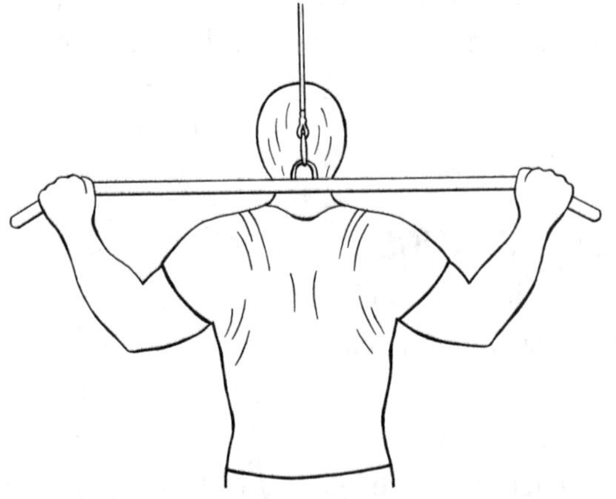

Fig. 10-11. Pull downs

NECK EXERCISES

Neck exercise machines provide the best way to gain strength without applying undue stress on your neck. These machines provide resistance during forward, backward, and side bending, and twisting of the neck (although twisting of the neck isn't recommended). Since not all health clubs or school weight rooms have these machines, if you don't have access to a neck machine, do the following isometric exercises. NEVER do neck bridges (Fig. 10-

12); this floor exercise is popular among wrestlers and football players.

How to perform exercises:

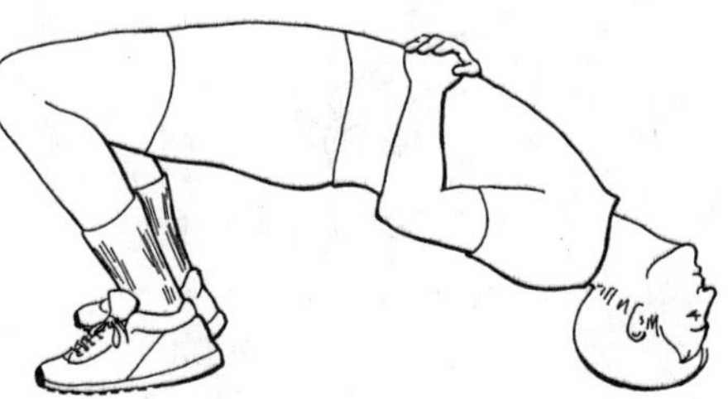

Fig. 10-12. Neck bridges

BACK OF NECK

Drop your head forward and place one hand on the back of your head. Push your head backward against your hand. Resist as much as possible while still moving the head slowly backward (Fig. 10-13).

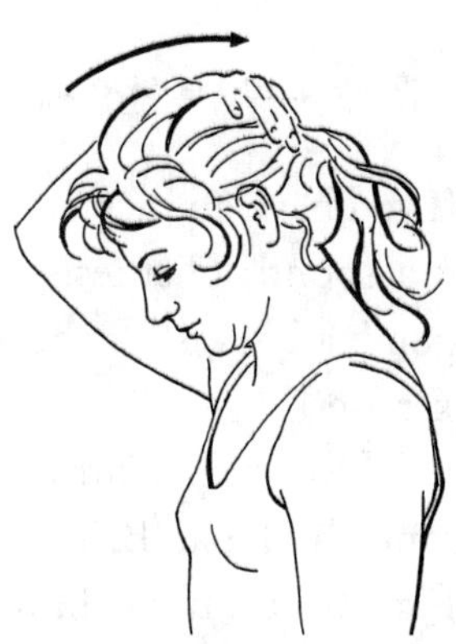

Fig. 10-13. Back of neck

FRONT OF THE NECK

Drop your head backward and place one hand on your forehead. Pull your head forward while applying resistance against your hand until your head has moved completely forward (Fig. 10-14).

SIDE OF NECK

Tilt your head all the way to the right side. With your right hand, reach over your head and apply resistance by pushing your head to the left. Once your head is at midline of your body, pull your head back to the right or away from the midline while applying resistance with your head. Repeat this exercise on the left side (Fig. 10-15).

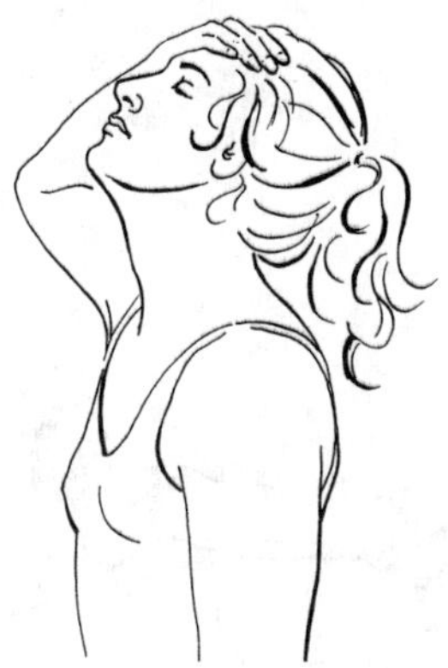

Fig. 10-14. Front of neck

HIP FLEXOR MUSCLES

HANGING KNEE RAISES/LEG LIFT

This exercise works both the abdominal and the hip flexor muscles. It is normal to have a forward curve in the low back, and this exercise will help to maintain that curvature.

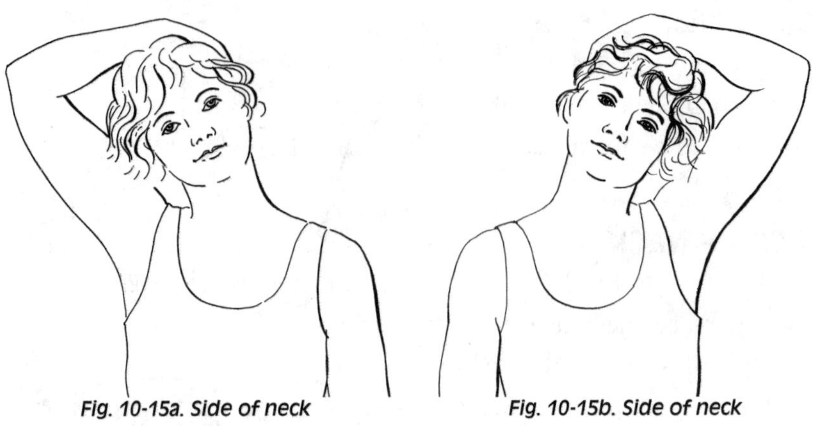

Fig. 10-15a. Side of neck

Fig. 10-15b. Side of neck

(If you have an increased forward curve—swayback—in the low back or a spondylolisthesis, do not perform this exercise. If you have a spondylolysis, seek the advice of your doctor before performing this exercise.)

How to perform exercise: This exercise is best done by hanging from a high bar. Bring your legs forward without bending your knees (Fig. 10-16). If you have difficulty with this exercise, bring your knees up toward your chest instead of doing straight-leg lifts (Fig. 10-17).

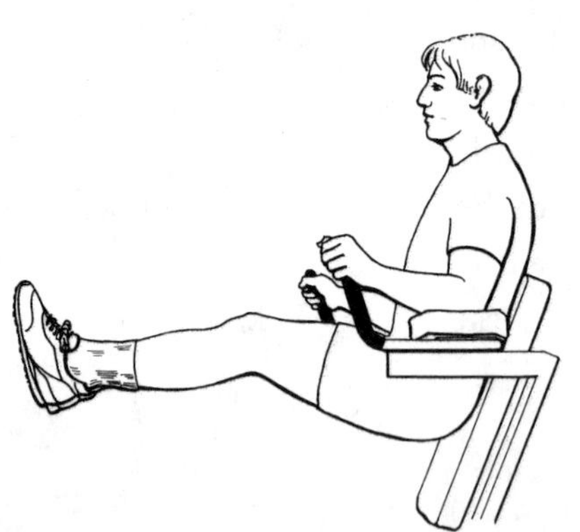

Fig. 10-16. Hanging leg lifts

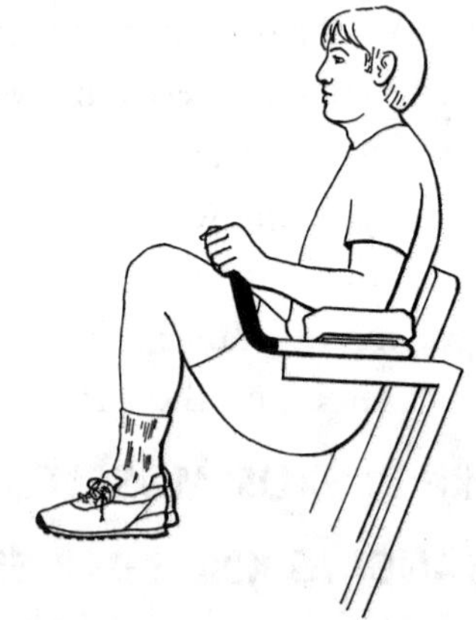

Fig. 10-17. Hanging knee raises (knee to chest)

LEG-STRAIGHTENING EXERCISES

Most people do front thigh exercises using a barbell. These exercises are called squats and lunges and can be classified as multijoint because they involve the knee and hip joints. The only multijoint exercise of the legs that I recommended is the lunge. Based on my experience as a weight-training instructor, there are several problems with using multijoint lower body exercises with a barbell. Even when you use good form, you have a chance of becoming off-balanced and of possibly straining your body. Problems can also occur when you load the barbell, especially since this is usually done with the barbell on the floor. Most of the students I've seen (even after they've been instructed not to) tend to bend forward and twist their body when loading weights on the barbell. There are many ways to do squats (front, hack, bench, rack, power rack), all of which include forward bending of the body while in the standing position and apply unnecessary stress to the low back (Fig. 10-18).

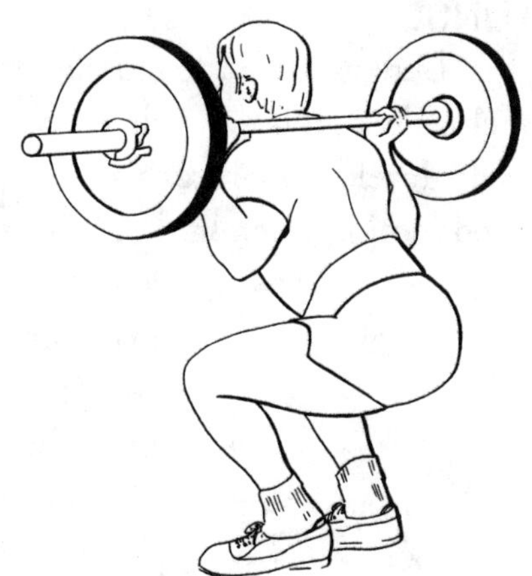

Fig. 10-18. Squats

It's best to avoid squats and concentrate on single-joint machines that better isolate specific muscle groups in the front thigh, back of the thigh, and back of the lower leg.

KNEE EXTENSORS

Knee extensors work the front thigh muscles, which are extremely important in maintaining proper posture and when lifting objects. As mentioned earlier, when lifting objects, never lean forward but always squat, bending your knees while keeping your back straight. Having strong front thigh muscles will enable you to lift with your legs for a longer period without your muscles getting tired. People have a

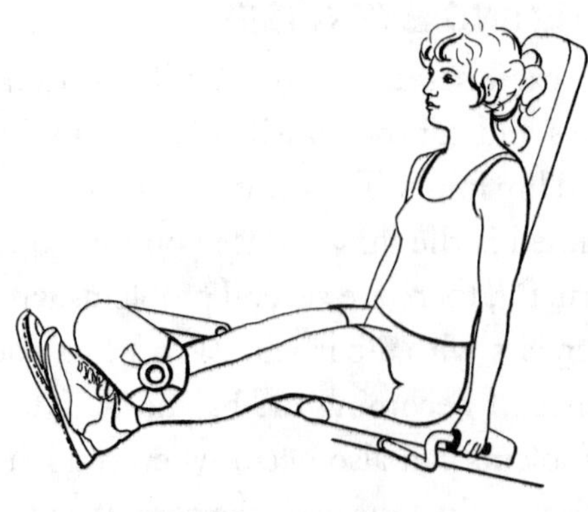

Fig. 10-19. Knee extensors

tendency when lifting objects to bend their back when their thigh muscles are weak or tired.

How to perform exercise: Knee extensors are performed on a knee extension machine. While in a seated position, place your feet under the padded bar. Pull your legs up until they are fully extended, then return to starting position (Fig. 10-19).

LUNGES

Lunges work the muscles of both the front thighs and the buttocks. These muscles help to maintain an erect posture and are often underdeveloped. Since this is an awkward exercise, make sure you have good footing when lifting. It is best to wear a flat and wide-base athletic shoe to gain extra stability. In addition, to maintain your stability and to help protect your knees, bend your knees only one third of their normal movement.

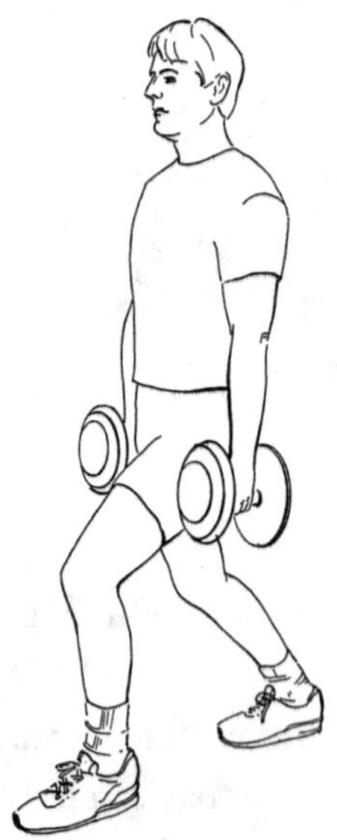

Fig. 10-20. Lunges

How to perform exercise: When lifting the dumbbells from the rack, stand directly facing the weights so that you do not twist and lean when picking up the weights. In a standing position, place your feet shoulder width. While holding a dumbbell in each hand, take a step forward, making sure your foot isn't placed in or out but is held straight ahead. Once your knees are bent about one third of their normal movement, return to the starting position. To help maintain proper posture and balance, keep your eyes focused on an object directly in front of you during the lunge. When pulling yourself back up, make sure to breathe out slowly. Repeat with other leg (Fig. 10-20).

INNER AND UPPER THIGHS

LEG PUSH

How to perform exercise: Standing with your body sideways to pulley machine, hook your outside foot into the ankle strap. Push your leg away from your body. Maintain your balance by holding onto a bar or your partner's shoulder and keep your back as straight as possible. Face the opposite direction and repeat the exercise with the opposite leg (Fig. 10-21).

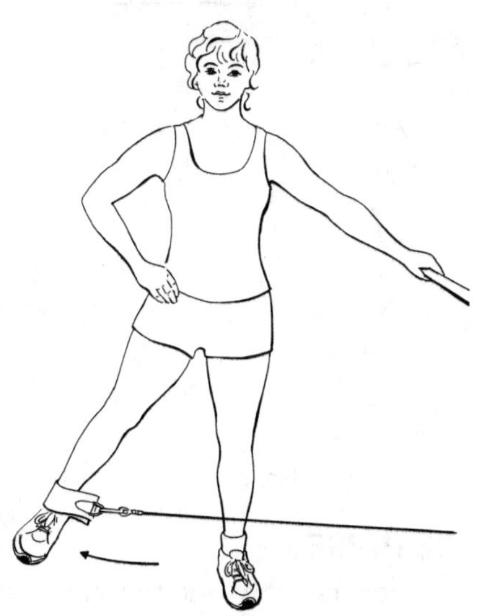

Fig. 10-21. Leg push

LEG PULLS

How to perform exercise: This exercise is best done with the help of a partner. Standing with your body sideways to pulley machine, hook your inside foot into the ankle strap. Maintain your balance by holding onto your partner's shoulder or a bar. Pull your leg toward the midline of your body. Your partner's main objective is to help you maintain your balance and help you keep your back straight as possible. Face the opposite direction and repeat the exercise with the opposite leg (Fig. 10-22).

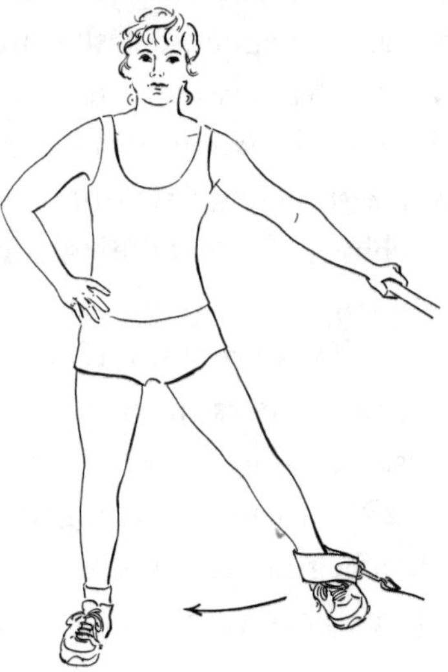

Fig. 10-22. Leg pulls

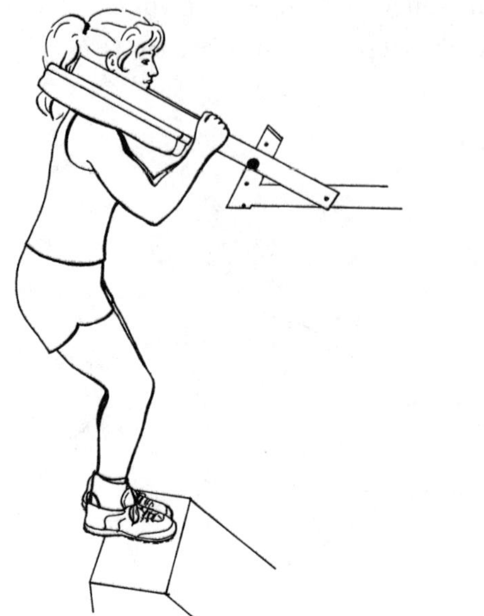

Fig. 10-23a. Toe raises

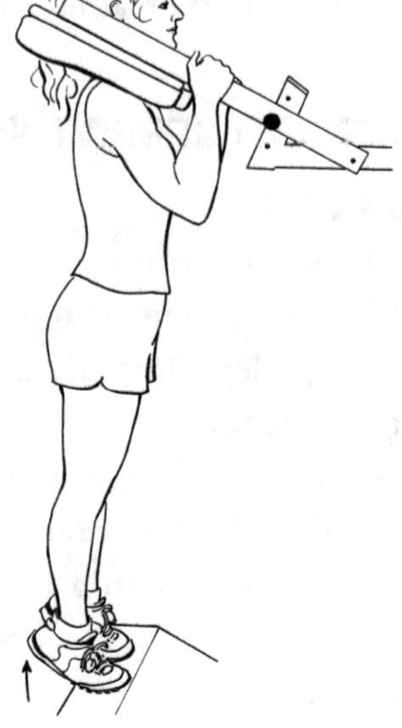

Fig. 10-23b. Toe raises

TOE RAISES

Toe raises work the calf muscles and can be done without weights. All you need is a block of wood and you can strengthen your calf muscles, although it's best to use weights, because the calf muscles are strong muscles that are usually able to lift more than your body weight. Most weight rooms and health clubs have a calf machine, although I recommend using dumbbells. If dumbbells can't provide you with enough weight, use a machine. If possible, use the sitting machine instead of the standing calf machine. This way, you won't load your back with weight.

How to perform exercise: Standing on the edge of a block with calf machine resting on your shoulders, slowly lift until you are on your toes, then slowly lower your feet until your heels touch the floor (Fig. 10-23). Be careful when going from a squatting to a standing position when beginning this exercise. Never round your back when standing. Always keep your back straight.

LEG CURLS

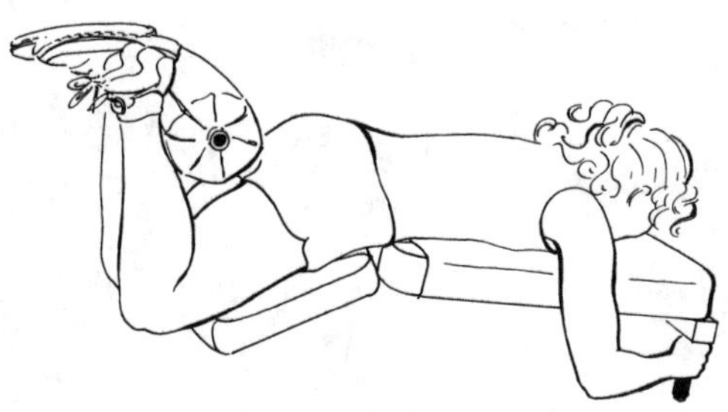

Fig. 10-24. Leg curls

The leg curl exercise works the muscles in the back of the thigh. Because most individuals have tight muscles in the back of the thigh, I recommend that the last leg exercise be leg curls. Since the front thigh muscles are stronger than the back thigh muscles, leg curls should always be done with a lower weight than the weight used in the knee extensor exercise.

How to perform exercise: Lie on your stomach on the leg curl machine. Place your legs under the pads of the machine. Bend your knees as far as you can but not more than about 100 degrees. Return to starting position (Fig. 10-24).

SHOULDERS, ARMS, AND CHEST

This weight-training workout places primary emphasis on the back, abdominal, and neck muscles. Secondary emphasis is on the leg muscles. The least emphasis is on the shoulders, arms, and chest muscles. The opposite is common among many weight lifters, who primarily emphasize the shoulders, arms, and chest while often neglecting the other parts of their body.

Since it is necessary to put more emphasis on the development of the muscles on the back side of the body (with the exception of the front thigh and abdominal muscles), you should do the shoulders, front arms muscles, and chest last in your weight-lifting routine.

Shoulders

The major shoulder muscle has three parts, all of which can be worked in the following exercise, called the overhead press. The overhead press can be done on a machine or with a barbell or dumbbells. It is best to sit rather than stand during this exercise. Make sure not to arch your low back when lifting.

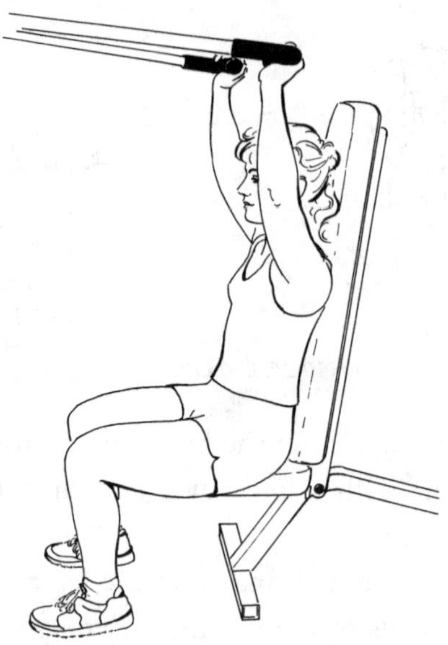

Fig. 10-25. Overhead press

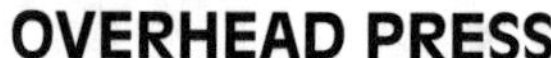

OVERHEAD PRESS

How to perform exercise: Sitting on a stool or padded seat, grab the bars and fully extend your arms above your head. Slowly lower the bar until you reach the starting position. Keep your eyes focused straight ahead so you won't tilt or lift your head (Fig. 10-25).

Arms

When carrying a load in your hands, always hold the load close to your body so as to place less stress on your back. Sufficient arm strength and muscle endurance will also help you to place less stress on your back when lifting or carrying objects.

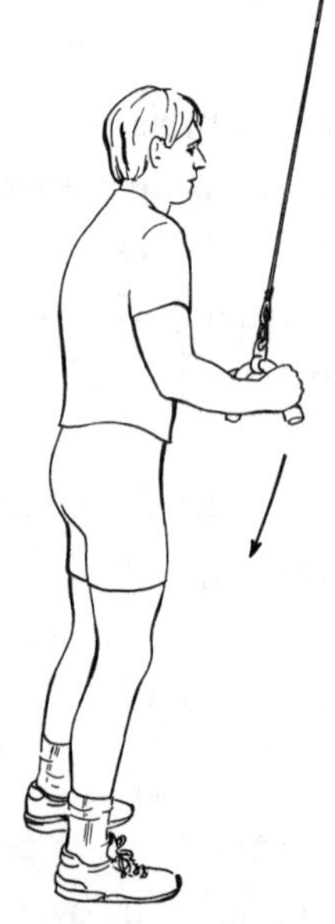

Fig. 10-26. Push-downs

Back of the Arms (Triceps)

Although many exercises work your triceps muscle, triceps exercises that require you to be seated or bent forward aren't recommended. These exercises tend to place unneeded stress upon your low back. Instead, do the triceps exercise in a standing position.

PUSH-DOWNS

It is best to avoid barbells and dumbbells during this exercise, since it is safer to do it on a machine.

How to perform exercise: Face the machine and grab the bar, keeping your elbows tight to the sides of your body. Push the bar down until your arms are completely straight. Make sure to stand straight and not to bend your upper body forward (Fig. 10-26).

FRONT OF THE ARMS

The front of the arm is developed by doing curl exercises. It is best to use a curl bar instead of a barbell or dumbbells when doing curls. A curl bar puts less stress upon the forearm muscles during this exercise, thus helping to prevent injury. A curl bar will also allow you to use more weight during this exercise. Always do curls in a standing position. Make sure not to arch your back when lifting. Doing preacher curls in a sitting position, where you perform this curl with your arms away from and in front of your body on a padded surface, should be avoided. This type of curl places unneeded stress to your neck and upper back.

CURLS

How to perform exercise: Grip the curl bar (Fig. 10-27) with your palms facing upward and your hands shoulder width apart. Lift your hands upwards toward your

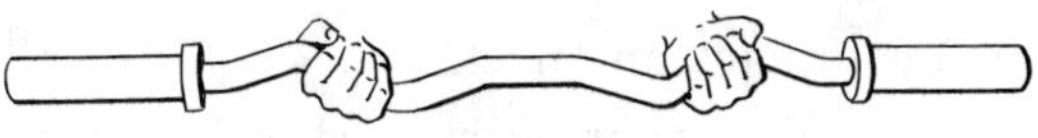

Fig. 10-27. Curl bar

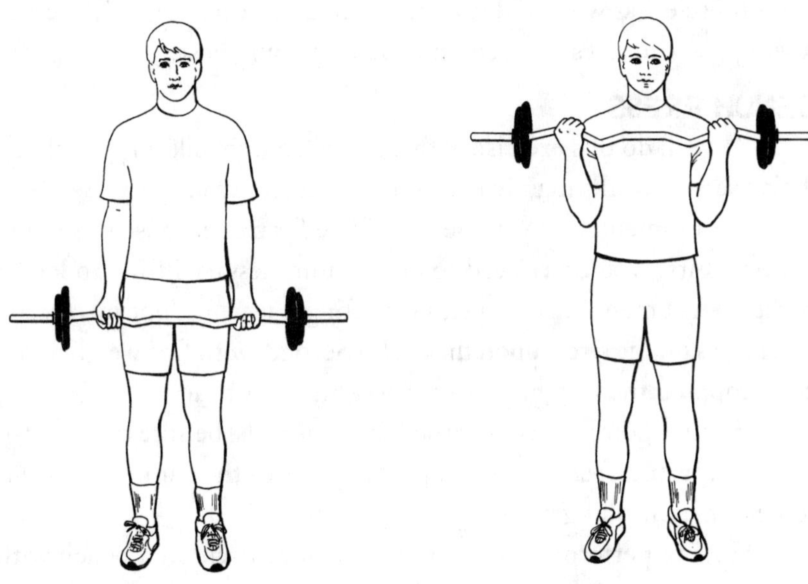

Fig. 10-28a. Curls

Fig. 10-28b. Curls

chest while keeping your spine straight. Slowly lower bar to starting position (Fig. 10-28).

Chest

The chest muscle can be divided into upper, middle, and lower parts. Since each part has muscle fibers that run in different directions, it will take three exercises to fully develop your chest.

When doing your chest exercises, never arch your back or your neck. It is common to see many weight lifters arch their backs when doing these exercises. Please don't fall into this habit. Do not bounce the weight off your chest either, because this can injure your chest bones and internal organs. Make sure to stretch your chest muscles as part of your regular workout. Contracted chest muscles can cause rounded shoulders. This improper posture places unneeded stress upon your back and neck.

Working your chest muscles involves multiple-joint exercises, which means you will be using two or more muscle groups when doing these exercises. This is also true of the pull-down exercise, which will strengthen the lower chest muscles as well as the back. Since the lower chest muscle was worked during the pull-down exercise, only the following two exercises are recommended for your chest.

BENCH PRESS

You can do this exercise with a barbell, dumbbells, or a machine. This exercise works mainly the middle chest muscle.

I recommend that you use a machine for this exercise for several reasons. First, you don't need to do any unnecessary lifting to load a barbell. (As I mentioned earlier, such lifting is usually done incorrectly and places undue stress upon the back.) Second, with free weights, you risk dropping the weight on your chest, neck, or head.

If you're going to use a barbell or dumbbells, be sure to have two spotters (partners) stationed at opposite ends of the bar or dumbbells to help in controlling the weight as you lift.

How to perform exercise: Lying on your back on a bench with your feet on the floor, grab the handles on the machine with your palms facing upward. Lift the weight until your arms are straight, then return to starting position. Your back should remain flat on the bench throughout the exercise (Fig. 10-29). **Never arch your low back when doing a bench press** (Fig. 10-30). Sharp and sudden contraction during a bench press can lead to injury and should be avoided. Lift smoothly and without jerking.

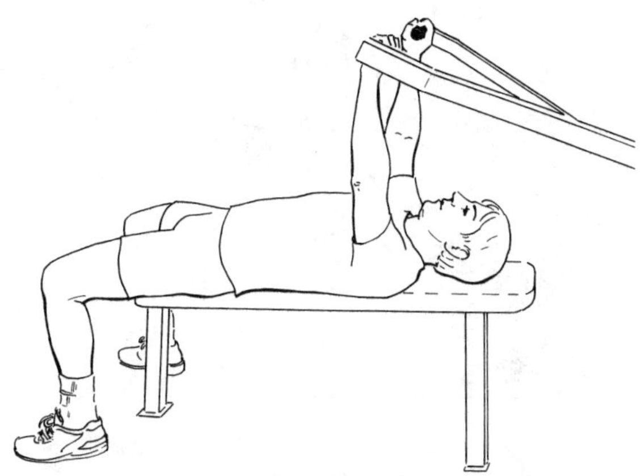

Fig. 10-29. Bench press

INCLINE BENCH PRESS

This exercise is similar to the bench press except that you are either standing or sitting on an incline bench. Also, with the incline bench press, you will lift the weight at a 45-degree angle rather than perpendicular to your chest. It is best for your back to use an incline bench that allows you to stand.

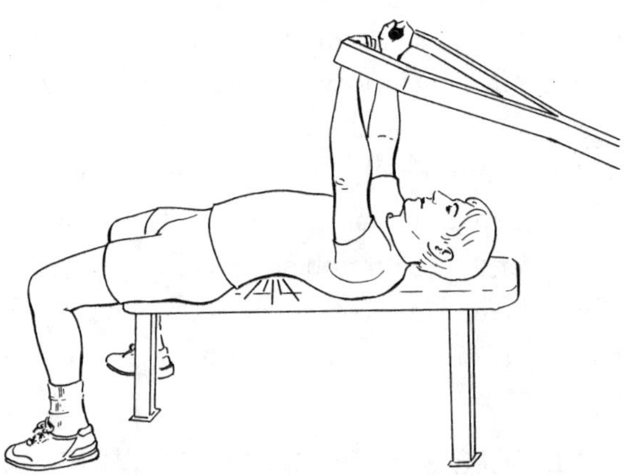

Fig. 10-30. Incorrect bench press

This exercise works the front shoulders and upper chest muscles. It can be done with a barbell, dumbbells, or a machine. Some machines simulate this lift and are sometimes found in local gyms and health clubs. If your weight room has this machine, use it. If you use a barbell or dumbbells, make sure to have two spotters.

How to perform exercise: With your back against the incline bench, grab the handles on the machine with your palms upward in starting position. Lift upward until your arms are straight then return to starting position (Fig. 10-31). Your back should remain **flat** on the bench throughout the exercise. As with the bench press, **never arch your low back when lifting.**

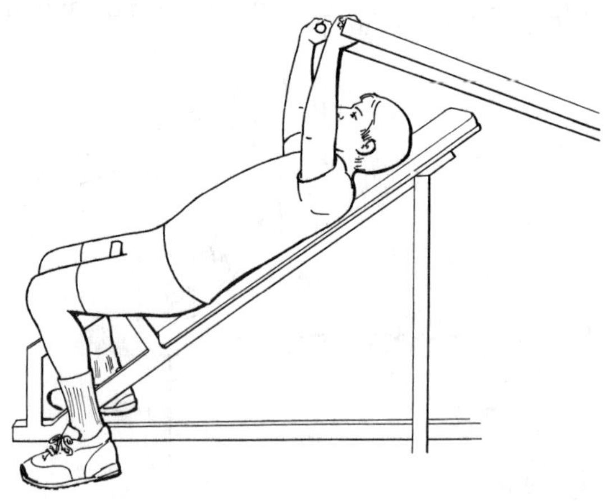

Fig. 10-31. Incline bench press

If you're lifting with a barbell or dumbbells, it is important that you lift toward the ceiling. If you lift the weight out in front of your body, you could injure your back and shoulders. Upon finishing, have the spotters grab the barbell or dumbbells. Do not lower the equipment to the ground yourself. The spotters can then return the barbell or dumbbells to the rack. It's better to use dumbbells rather then a barbell. Dumbbells are usually preloaded in most weight rooms and stored on a rack, while a barbell needs to be loaded for both you and your partners.

MUSCLE SORENESS FOLLOWING WEIGHT TRAINING

If you become sore after your weight-training routine, you have lifted too hard. Soreness is a result of waste buildup in your muscles or possible over stretched or even torn tissue, both of which should be avoided. Always remember that your goal in exercising is to reduce the risk factors related to back pain.

STEROIDS

I know there will always be some unethical athletes who will take steroids to increase their size, strength, or speed. That is wrong. The majority of people who take steroids do it to "improve" their appearance. I'm always amazed that a person will ruin his or her health (see Table 10-3) or risk dying at an early age so that he or she can, in theory, have a massive, good-looking body. GET REAL!

Having respect for your body is good, but using destructive, illegal drugs shows anything but respect for your body or your health. Use your desire to look good by exercising regularly and naturally. In the long run, you will be healthier and will feel better about yourself. If you still don't want an average build, spend extra time lifting weights to build your muscles. Above all, stay away from steroids. They're bad news!

TABLE 10-3
HEALTH CONDITIONS RELATED TO STEROID USE

Acne	Kidney disease
Bad breath	Liver disease
Baldness	Nose bleeds
Cancer	Oily skin
Heart disease	Shrunken breasts
High blood pressure	Shrunken testicles
Impotence	Stunted growth
Infertility	Uncontrollable anger

CONCLUSION

If you wish to gain more information on weight training, see the recommended reading list in Appendix A. The books I recommend were written by experts in the field of physical education and will provide you with the training effects, physiology, and general knowledge regarding weight training.

The following chapter discusses how to stay motivated by changing unhealthy actions into healthy habits. Simple changes in your lifestyle are all that you need to develop and maintain a healthy back and body. Many of us know we should exercise, but we don't because many of us don't know how to introduce and maintain the necessary lifestyle changes. The following chapter presents ideas on how to make these changes easier.

CHAPTER II

Motivation

GOOD HEALTH IS DETERMINED in large part by living a healthy lifestyle in which you control your health by choosing healthy habits and eliminating unhealthy actions and behavior. Unfortunately, only 20 percent of adult Americans currently choose to participate in an exercise program that will produce health-related benefits. Another 40 percent of adults participate in leisure activities that don't provide enough benefit to produce a fit and healthy body. The remaining 40 percent of adult Americans are couch potatoes and don't exercise at all.

According to many fitness experts, what prevents most people from participating in an exercise program isn't their ability but their attitudes and behavior. By having certain self-perceptions, people develop beliefs that are counterproductive to starting and maintaining an exercise program. Many people believe they are too old, too chubby, or too busy to work out. Others may suffer from low self-esteem and possibly feel that they aren't athletic or capable of being physically active. Then there is the type-A personality, who starts an exercise program with a gung-ho, win-at-all-costs, no-pain, no-gain attitude and who, after a few weeks, either gets burned out or develops an injury, preventing further activity. Whether from procrastination or a simple dislike for exercise, a person's behavior limits the person from maintaining an exercise program.

Don't kid yourself. A healthy behavior is made, not born. You can develop behavior to fit your needs and aspirations. What you will need for developing a healthy behavior are goal setting, motivation, and social support. To train yourself physically, you will need to visualize yourself as a physically active person. The more you see yourself as physically active, the more likely you are to break down some of your inappropriate self-beliefs and to want to exercise. Therefore, most people who wish to physically train will need to mentally train as well.

UNDERSTANDING MOTIVATION

Motivation consists of two critical elements: intensity and direction. Intensity is related to the amount of effort given to attain a certain goal, while direction deals with the reason a person chooses to pursue or avoid pursuing a certain goal. To have successful direction, a person must feel that a certain goal will provide or achieve a personal need that he or she perceives to be important. The more important this goal is perceived to be, the more direction and intensity the person will apply to it.

You must therefore learn to perceive your health as being important. Many of us take our health for granted. As a result, our unhealthy habits eventually create health problems. Not only can these health problems affect your quality of life, but they can also shorten your life. Just knowing that not exercising, smoking, and eating a high-fat diet are detrimental to your health isn't enough. You must reinforce the positive aspects of good health and work to incorporate healthy habits into your lifestyle. Whether you are elderly, disabled, or simply unfit, exercise can help to give you a feeling of well-being. Exercise has been found to lower depression and anxiety, give you more energy and self-confidence, and help you to feel better about yourself, all of which help to improve your productivity and quality of life.

Wouldn't it be wonderful if the benefits of exercise could be made into a pill? Everyone would be addicted to it. But in reality, you are responsible for developing your own sense of well-being and quality of life. The best way to do so is to first establish goals.

Goal Setting

Goals give you a sense of direction. If the goal is also perceived to be important, it will give you some intensity. To become good at goal setting, you have to implement a set of basic rules. First, you need to establish specific, realistic, challenging, short-term performance-oriented goals. By making your goals as specific as possible, you're directing your behavior to a specific mode of action. This will lead to more success, since you will know definitely what action is required to accomplish your goals.

Finding realistic yet challenging goals is often the most difficult part of fitness goal setting. Exercise programs that are perceived as hard and that involve activities of greater intensity are associated with significantly lower adherence. The best way that you can find a comfortable yet challenging workout is to check your pulse rate and assess how you feel during and after a workout, as discussed in Chapter 9.

Second, never set a goal based on the OUTCOME of your fitness training, such as having a trim physique, swimming a mile in 20 minutes, or bench pressing 300 pounds. If you concentrate on the end product, you will get frustrated easier and may quit because the goal seems unrealistic. Planning with short-term goals will make the activity seem easier and more rewarding. This will create a greater adherence, which in the long run will help you accomplish your long-term goals.

Third, you should develop short-term performance goals daily. After you have found your pulse rate and determined how you feel, you will be ready to set a daily plan for your workout. In the morning, you will decide when, where, what, and how you will perform your exercise. In deciding when, you will need to determine the exact time you will work out. This forces you to check your daily schedule and decide when you're able to make time for your fitness program. Now that you have decided that exercise is a primary goal in your daily lifestyle, your fitness program should take a high priority in your daily activities.

Next you will need to determine what type of exercise you will perform each day. For example, if after your warm up you decide to weight train, you need to know whether you will work your upper or lower body. If you decide to do some conditioning, you need to know whether it will be cycling, walking, stair climbing, etc. Remember, too, to end your workout with a cool-down routine.

You've already read about how to warm up and cool down, weight train, and condition your body. It's important also that you use a workout log, which will help you to keep track of your progress and the exercises you will do and their sequence. These records also provide positive feedback and reinforcement of your goals and workouts. The workout logs are in Appendix D.

MOTIVATION AND SOCIAL SUPPORT

As previously mentioned, research has shown that one of the major ingredients to maintaining an exercise program is to have a workout that you perceive as being easy. Therefore, when starting out, do less than you think you can and progress only after you have shown that you can follow an exercise routine within your schedule. This will give you a sense of accomplishment and help you to achieve your new exercise commitment rather than cause you to burn out shortly after starting.

It is also important to find ways to make your exercise fun. You can accomplish this by choosing a conditioning exercise that you find enjoyable. Obviously, the more you enjoy a certain activity, the more likely you are to stick with it. You also may wish to vary your activities in your conditioning routine or vary the days that you lift and condition. Another way to enjoy your exercise routine is to exercise with others. Exercise can be a great way to break down barriers and meet others who share your exercise goals yet also want to socialize.

Many experts believe there are two distinct ways to motivate yourself to accomplish your goals. The first is intrinsic motivation, which comes from you and not from any outside sources. Because you love the sport or activity or wish to become competent or successful at it, you try harder to develop the needed tasks. Also, since you're satisfied with the activities, you rarely miss a workout. These are forms of intrinsic motivation that are self-started.

Extrinsic motivation, on the other hand, comes from outside sources that are used to help you achieve your goals. For example, you may want to exercise because you wish to receive recognition through an award or a plaque. Or perhaps you wish to achieve a certain amount of mileage in your conditioning workout in a certain amount of time. If this is the case, then you are seeking an outside source to help you stay motivated.

Of course, it is best to have both forms of motivation working for you. Ideally, it would be nice if we all were internally motivated, but most of us need some form of outside help. If you're fortunate enough to work for an employer who has a worksite exercise facility or will pay for your health club membership, don't be shy. Take advantage of such an opportunity. Many employers add incentive by lowering their employees' health insurance premiums or awarding extra vacation days for participating regularly in an exercise program. Everyone should be so lucky!

To develop a commitment and a sense of satisfaction to an exercise program, sign a workout contract and use a reward system. That's right. You need to sign a contract and have it witnessed by a friend or even by an adversary (see Appendix D). You may wish to have in writing an agreed penalty if you don't stay committed to your workout. For example, you will agree to mow your friend's lawn for the next six months or walk your friend's dog four times a week for two months if you break your contract.

Your next move is to develop some kind of reward system based on your participation. It is best to give yourself small rewards on a weekly or monthly basis and a big reward on an annual basis. Since you should always reward yourself in a way that is conducive to developing a healthy body, rewarding yourself with a big dinner or a half gallon of ice cream at the end of the week isn't allowed. Try to be inventive and think of ways to make it fun and enjoyable.

This fitness program can produce health-related benefits only if you exercise regularly. Since participation is your primary objective, why not develop a reward system with this in mind. You might choose the following weekly exercise routine: (1) four days of weight lifting (two days to work your lower body and two days for your upper body), (2) three days of conditioning, and (3) seven days of warming up and cooling down (done before both weight lifting and conditioning). With this schedule, give yourself a point for each component of exercise that you participate in: possible four points for weight training, three for conditioning, and seven for your warm-up and cool-down routines. In addition, when you have completed all components of your workout schedule, give yourself an extra six points, thereby giving yourself 20 points for the week. Even if you fall short by two exercise sessions per week, you will still have 10 points.

Reward yourself after you have accumulated a certain number of points per week, per month, or per year. This is where the fun part begins. Let's say you get 80 points your first month and you reward yourself with a special purchase or by allowing yourself more time for a hobby. Don't spend all of your money or time on this first month's reward, because at the end of each succeeding month, you should have another reward, and at the end of one full year, you can give yourself a big reward, such as a recreational vacation.

Let's say that you have reached your goal of 900 points at the end of the year and now deserve a fun vacation. Remember to include your family and friends who, after all, have helped by allowing you time and encouraging you to exercise. Whatever your conditioning activity, a recreational vacation is waiting for you. If you like aerobic dancing, why not travel on a cruise ship where you also will have a weight-training room. How about bicycling along the Florida coast or through Yosemite Valley. You like the water. How about snorkeling in Hawaii. Maybe your reward is walking regularly at your favorite getaway spot. Whatever you choose, make sure it's something you enjoy.

Have fun in the future by staying active today. All you need is to make some simple changes and you will be on your way. You will find that your new attitude will be exciting and full of adventure. More important, you'll no longer take for granted your good health. In fact, you'll cherish it.

The more you work to develop a healthy behavior, the more likely you will succeed. May I recommend two books to help you stay motivated. You'll find the title of these books in the recommended reading list in Appendix A.

Conclusion

ONCE YOUR BACK, which normally is durable, strong, and pain free, has been injured or wear and tear has occurred, its tissue weakens. Unlike bone, which heals stronger when broken, torn muscle, disc, cartilage, or ligament tissue heals with less durable and elastic material. If left unchecked, this could lead to further impairment and pain.

This book has shown you how to lower your risk for back pain through exercising correctly, losing weight, eating properly, and improving your psychological health. As you now know, the best way to deal with back pain is to prevent it. If you minimize the known risks to your back and work to maintain your good health, you can help to prevent a bad back. An added benefit to this is the reduction in risk of cardiovascular disease and improvement in your overall health.

At last, you now have a complete guide to fight off the most common health complaint affecting working Americans. Back pain has reached epidemic proportions, creating far too much suffering. Yet until now, little, if any, information has been available to help individuals reduce the risk of back pain.

Why wait for a backache and other health impairments to develop and lower your quality of life? Take some control of your health and let the back-friendly workout help you to improve the function of your spine. This comprehensive workout and other back-building tips will allow you to be physically and mentally healthier with a minimal amount of time. Most of all, it will allow you to have fun by living an active lifestyle, and that's what living is all about!

Appendix A

RESOURCES

Back-Building Seminars

Conducted by Dr. Whitney, these seminars are open to businesses, educators, health-care professionals, and groups interested in preventive health. Participants will receive personal instruction and information on ways to prevent back pain and promote good health. For more information, write to Kat Hill Communications, PO Box 3044, Antioch, CA 94531.

Recommended Reading

Stretching:

Stretching
B. Anderson, Shelter Publications Inc., 1980.
The Book About Stretching
S. Solvenborn, Japan Publications Inc., 1985.

Weight Training:

Basic Weight Training
T. Fahey, Mayfield Publishing, 1989.
Weight Training Today
B. O'Conner, J. Simmons, P. O'Shea
West Publishing Co., 1989.
Weight Training for Women

T. Fahey, G. Hutchinson
Mayfield Publishing, 1992.

Conditioning:

Walking for Health
L. Seiger, J. Hesson
Wm. C Brown Publishers, 1990.
Learn how to get or stay in shape by walking as part of your total workout.

Swim for the Health of It
E.W. Maglischo, C.F. Brennan. Mayfield Publishing, 1985.
This book will teach you the proper mechanics and training procedures as they apply to swimming.

Ropics
K.M. Solis, Human Kinetics Publishers, 1992.
This book will teach you how to jump rope and train effectively.

Aqua Aerobics Today
C. Casten, West Publishing Co., 1994.
This complete book will be your resource for learning about water exercise. Proper equipment, water resistance, exercisers with special needs, and a lot more are taught in this book.

Basketball Skills and Drills
J. Krause, Human Kinetics Publishers, 1991.
Learn the basics of basketball and how to develop your skills.

Soccer
J.A. Luxbacher, Human Kinetics Publishers, 1991.
This self instruction guide allows you to learn the game and develop skills on your own.

The Aerobics Program for Total Well-Being
K.H. Cooper, Bantam Books, 1982.
Learn how conditioning and diet can affect your overall health.

Exercise Motivation:

Fitness Motivation
W.J. Rejeski, E. Kenney, Life Enhancement Publications, 1988.

Coaches' Guide to Sport Psychology
R. Martens, Human Kinetics Publishers, Inc., 1987.
Fitness Instruction:
Guidelines for Exercise Testing and Prescription, 5th ed.
American College of Sports Medicine,
Williams and Williams Publishing, 1995.
(800) 638-0672
Sitting Instruction:
Sitting on the Job
S.W. Donkin, Houghton Mifflin, 1989.
Learn how to survive the stresses of sitting. Instruction is given on how to adjust your workstation and chair in a back friendly manner.

Exercise and Diet Information Sources:
American College of Sports Medicine
P.O. Box 1440
Indianapolis, IN 46206-1440
(317) 637-9200
For information on how to select a health/fitness facility in your local area, send a self-addressed, stamped, business size envelop to ACSM Public Information Department. It will send you the free 12-page pamphlet titled "Health/Fitness Facilities Consumer Selection Guide." In addition, ACSM has numerous publications for the general public regarding health-related fitness. If you are interested in becoming a fitness instructor or wish to keep up on current information regarding exercise and sports medicine, call for membership.
The Aerobics and Fitness Association of America
15250 Ventura Blvd., Suite 310
Sherman Oaks, CA 91403
(800) 446-AFAA
AFAA has a consumer hotline to help you find a certified AFAA aerobics dance instructor in your area.

IDEA: International Association for Fitness Professionals
6190 Cornerstone Ct. E., Ste. 204
San Diego, CA 92121-3773
(800) 999-IDEA

If you have the money and desire, IDEA has a consumer hotline to help you find a certified personal fitness trainer in your area. A personal trainer can be helpful in seeking advice and motivation to start or continue the back-friendly workout.

American Dietetic Association
216 W. Jackson Blvd., Suite 800
Chicago, IL 60606
(800) 366-1655

The ADA will provide you with nutritional information on how to establish and maintain a proper diet. The above phone number will provide you with a registered dietician to answer your nutritional questions.

Information on how to stop smoking:

American Lung Association
1740 Broadway
New York, NY 10019-4374
(800) LUNG-USA

The ALA will provide you with the following information to help you quit smoking: self-help kits, seminars, and many other supplies. Some local chapters may supply videos and workbooks or support groups.

Finding an ergonomic specialist:

Human Factors and Ergonomics Society
P.O. Box 1369
Santa Monica, CA 90406
(310) 394-1811

This society publishes a consultants directory of ergonomic specialists who are trained in worksite evaluations. The directory sells for $35.00 plus shipping.

Supplies:

Mattresses

There are a number of mattress manufacturers, including King Koil, Ortho, Serta, and Springwall, to name a few. These manufacturers usually have a number of different mattress designs. When it comes to mattresses, you get what you pay for. It is therefore best to buy the top designs. If possible, wait for a sale, where it is not unusual to save up to 50%. I'm convinced that there isn't one manufacturer that makes the perfect bed for everyone. I therefore recommend when shopping for a new mattress that you actually lie on the bed to see which one feels most comfortable. Having a firm, comfortable top design mattress is what you want.

General Supplies

Relax The Back Store (National Franchise)
Headquarters
3355 Bee Cave Rd., Bldg. 7
Austin, TX 78746
(800) 290-BACK

This chain of stores offers a complete list of back-friendly supplies. For example, chairs, mattresses, pillows, supports, are available. Call to see if there is a store near you. If not, order by e-mail or possibly over the phone.

Information regarding proper body mechanics:

American Chiropractic Association
1701 Clarendon Blvd.
Arlington, VA 22209
(800) 368-3083

ACA has pamphlets on the proper way to lift, sit, stand, and maintain good posture. Information is also available on the dangers of taking steroids. Call for free catalog.

Ergonomic educational material:

Ergodyne Inc.

PO Box
St. Paul, Minn 22222
(800) 225-8238

Ergodyne has booklets available to the general public regarding practical ergonomic tips for office workers, and those exposed to repetitive trauma at work.

Periodicals

These periodicals will keep you current on the following back-friendly conditioning activities. Learn the proper techniques, ways to stay healthy, how to have fun, and much more.

The Walking Magazine
Customer Service Dept.
P.O. Box 56561
Boulder, CO 80322-6561
(800) 678-0881

Swim Magazine
P.O. Box 91870
Pasadena, CA 91109
(800) 538-9787

Sidekicks Soccer Magazine
19 West 21st St.
New York, NY 10010
(800) 938-5588

Slam Basketball Magazine
1115 Broadway
New York, NY 10010
(212) 807-7100

Recreational Vacations

Club Med
7975 N. Hayden Rd.
Scottsdale, AZ 85258
(800) 258-2633
Call for summer, winter, or cruise ship brochure.

Backroads Touring Co.
1515 5th St., Suite A110
Berkeley, CA 94710
(800) GO-ACTIVE or 462-2848
This company offers bicycle and walking tours throughout the world. Call for free catalog.

Appendix B

Before you look at the weight chart on the next page, determine the size of your body frame by measuring the circumference of your wrist. Then match your body frame to your height on the weight chart to determine your ideal weight.

Women:

Small	Medium	Large
less than 5 1/4"	5 1/4-6"	more than 6"

Men:

Small	Medium	Large
less than 6 1/4"	6 1/4-7"	more than 7"

Men

Height Feet	Inches	Small Frame	Medium Frame	Large Frame
5	2	128-134	131-141	138-150
5	3	130-136	133-143	140-153
5	4	132-138	135-145	142-156
5	5	134-140	137-148	144-160
5	6	136-142	139-151	146-164
5	7	138-145	142-154	149-168
5	8	140-148	145-157	152-172
5	9	142-151	148-160	155-176
5	10	144-154	151-163	158-180
5	11	146-157	154-166	161-184
6	0	149-160	157-170	164-188
6	1	152-164	160-174	168-192
6	2	155-168	164-178	172-197
6	3	158-172	167-182	176-202
6	4	162-176	171-187	181-207

Source: Metropolitan Life Insurance Company.

Women

Height Feet	Inches	Small Frame	Medium Frame	Large Frame
4	10	102-111	109-121	118-131
4	11	103-113	111-123	120-134
5	0	104-115	113-126	122-137
5	1	106-118	115-129	125-140
5	2	108-121	118-132	128-143
5	3	111-124	121-135	131-147
5	4	114-127	124-138	134-151
5	5	117-130	127-141	137-155
5	6	120-133	130-144	140-159
5	7	123-136	133-147	143-163
5	8	126-139	136-150	146-167
5	9	129-142	139-153	149-170
5	10	132-145	142-156	152-173
5	11	135-148	145-159	155-176
6	0	138-151	148-162	158-179

Source: Metropolitan Life Insurance Company.

The table lists weight in pounds for men and women, age 25 to 59, in indoor clothing. Weights are according to height, including one-inch heels, with five pounds of clothing for men and three pounds of clothing for women.

Appendix C

CONNIE AND OTIS BEFORE AND AFTER SCORES

Refer to complete questionnaire in Chapter 4 for examples on how numbers are computed.

Connie Before Back Building

INDIVIDUAL RISK FACTORS

1. Age

35-55	56 & up	18-34
20	15	5

Points 20

2. Smoking
Cigarettes per Day

1-5	6-10	11-20	21 or more
5	10	20	30

Points 0

3. Exercise

If you already participate in the back-friendly workout, no points will be added to the next three questions. However, if you don't participate in this workout program, you'll need to add the appropriate points. If you currently stretch, weight train, or participate in a conditioning workout, finish reading this book before answering the following three questions. If you aren't doing any of the above activities, go ahead and answer questions A, B, and C.

A. Do you participate in a regular full-body weight-training workout two to three times a week?

Yes	No
5	10

Points 10

B. Do you participate in a regular full-body stretching routine four to five times a week?

Yes	No
5	10

Points 10

C. Do you participate in a regular conditioning workout at least three times a week for about 20-30 minutes?

Yes	No
5	10

Points 10

4. Do you always wear a seat belt while in a motor vehicle?

Yes	No
0	5

Points 0

5. Are you tall?

Men:

5'10"- 6'0"	over 6'0"- 6'2"
1 pt.	2 pts.
over 6'2"- 6'4"	over 6'4"
3 pts.	4 pts.

Points 0

Women:

5'5"- 5'7"	over 5'7"- 5'9"
1 pt.	2 pts.
over 5'9"- 5'11"	over 5'11"
3 pts.	4 pts.

Points 2

6. Body frame size

Women:

Small	Medium	Large
less than 5 1/4″	5 1/4-6″	more than 6″

Men:

Small	Medium	Large
less than 6 1/4″	6 1/4-7″	more than 7″

Overweight by

< 10 %	10-19%	20-29%	30-39 %	40 % or >
1 pt.	2 pts.	3 pts.	4 pts.	5 pts.

Points 2

TABLE 4-2

RISK FOR LIFTING AND CARRYING AT HOME

TIME

	1 hour or less	Occasional 1-2 hours	Intermittent 2-4 hours	Frequent 4-6 hours	Constant 6-8 hours
5-10% Minimal	1	1.5	2	~~3~~	3.5
11-25% Light	1.5	~~2~~	2-3	3-4	4-5
26-50% Moderate	~~2~~	2-3	4-5	4-6	5-7
51-75% Heavy	~~3~~	3-4	4-6	7-10	10-15
76% & up Very Heavy	~~3.5~~	4-5	5-7	10-15	20-30
Points	8.5	2		3	

Total Points 13.5

TABLE 4-3
MOVEMENTS DURING NONWORK ACTIVITIES

(Cross off the appropriate point box)

Activity	1 hr.	2 hrs.	3 hrs.	4 hrs.	5 hrs.	6 hrs.	7 hrs.	8 hrs.
	Number of hours per day							
Twisting	3	4	5	6	7	8	9	10
Bending forward	2	3	4	5	6	7	8	9
Reaching outward	2	3	4	5	6	7	8	9
Bending backward	1	2	3	4	5	6	7	8
Sitting	1	2	3	4	5	6	7	8
Driving	1	2	3	4	5	6	7	8
One-sided movements	1	2	3	4	5	6	7	8
Pushing & pulling	0	0	1	2	3	4	5	6
Standing	0	0	0	0	0	1	2	3
Average Daily Points	5	6	4					

* Driving includes, noncommute driving of cars, trucks, or recreational vehicles.

Total Points 15

DETERMINING ADDITIONAL RISK FOR WOMEN

A. Are you a Causcasian woman?

Yes	No
1	0

B. As a child and a young adult, did (do) you have a diet low in dairy products (milk, cheese, etc.)?

Yes	No
1	0

C. Do you consume a high-protein diet? Food consists of carbohydrates, protein, and fats. If you consume above 15% of your total food intake from protein, the answer is yes. Protein is found in meats, fish, beans, nuts, and dairy products.

Yes	No
1	0

D. Do you consume large amounts of caffeine (more than 4 cups of coffee, tea or cola beverages per day)?

Yes	No
1	0

Total Osteoporosis Points 3

2. Multiple pregnancies:
Number of Pregnancies

2	3	4	above 5
1	2	4	5

Total Points 4

Your total individual risk: points 89.5

OCCUPATIONAL RISK FACTORS

TABLE 4-4

RISK FOR LIFTING AND CARRYING AT WORK

TIME

	1 hour or less	Occasional 1-2 hours	Intermittent 2-4 hours	Frequent 4-6 hours	Constant 6-8 hours
5-10% Minimal	1	1.5	2	3	~~3.5~~
11-25% Light	1.5	2	2-3	~~3-4~~	4-5
26-50% Moderate	2	2-3	~~4-5~~	4-6	5-7
51-75% Heavy	3	~~3-4~~	4-6	7-10	10-15
76% & up Very Heavy	~~3.5~~	4-5	5-7	10-15	20-30
Points	3.5	3	4	4	3.5

Total Points 18

TABLE 4-5

MOVEMENTS AT WORK

(Cross off the appropriate point box)

Activity	Number of hours per day 1 hr.	2 hrs.	3 hrs.	4 hrs.	5 hrs.	6 hrs.	7 hrs.	8 hrs.
Twisting	3	~~4~~	5	6	7	8	9	10
Bending forward	2	3	4	~~5~~	6	7	8	9
Reaching outward	2	3	4	~~5~~	6	7	8	9
Bending backward	1	2	3	4	5	6	7	8
Sitting	1	2	3	4	5	6	7	8
Driving*	1	2	3	4	5	6	7	8
Vibrational forces (e.g. jackhammer)	1	2	3	4	5	6	7	8
One-sided movements	1	2	3	~~4~~	5	6	7	8
Pushing & pulling	0	~~0~~	1	2	3	4	5	6
Standing	0	0	0	0	0	1	2	~~3~~
Average Daily Points		4		14				3

* Driving includes, cars, trucks, forklifts, or other moving equipment, both at work and commuting.

Total Points 21

Your total occupation risk: Points 39

RECREATIONAL RISK FACTORS

TABLE 4-6
RECREATIONAL ACTIVITIES

	Frequency				
	Minimal	Occasional	Regular		
Activity	1-3 month	1-2 a week	3-7 a week	Annual Amount	
HOCKEY	.2	.6	.8	X	=
RODEO RIDING	.2	.6	.8	X	=
FOOTBALL/ RUGBY	.2	.6	.8	X	=
GOLF	.1	.5	.6	X	=
GYMNASTICS	.1	.5	.6	X	=
BACKPACKING	.1	.4	.5	X	=
JAVELIN THROWING	.1	.4	.5	X	=
RACQUETBALL	.1	.4	.5	X	=
BOWLING	.1	.4	.5	X 52	= 20.8
SQUASH	.1	.4	.5	X	=
HANDBALL	.1	.4	.5	X	=
ROWING	.1	.4	.5	X	=
JOGGING	.1	.4	.5	X	=
CROSS-COUNTRY SKIING	.1	.4	.5	X	=
WRESTLING	.1	.4	.5	X	=
BASEBALL/SOFTBALL	.1	.4	.5	X	=
TENNIS	.1	.4	.5	X	=

Your total recreational risk: Points 20.8

PSYCHOLOGICAL RISK FACTORS

The following questions deal with how your behavior may play a role in the development of back pain:

1. How would you describe your ability to tolerate pain?

Normal	Above normal	Below normal
0 pts	-3 pts	+3 pts

Points 0

2. Do you have a high level of emotional stress at home or at work?

Yes	No
+3 pts	0 pts

Points 3

3. Do you experience anxiety frequently at work or while at home?

Yes	No
+3 pts	0 pts

Points 0

Your total psychological risk: Points 3

Use the following chart to total your points in each risk category.

Your Total Points

Individual risk total	89.5
Occupational risk total	39.0
Recreational risk total	20.8
Psychological risk total	3.0
Total Points	152.3

Guidelines for Back Pain

Some risk	Moderate risk	High risk
< 50 pts.	50-100 pts.	> 100 pts.

Connie After Back Building

INDIVIDUAL RISK FACTORS

1. Age

35-55	56 & up	18-34
20	15	5

Points 20

2. Smoking
Cigarettes per Day

1-5	6-10	11-20	21 or more
5	10	20	30

Points 0

3. Exercise

If you already participate in the back-friendly workout, no points will be added to the next three questions. However, if you don't participate in this workout program, you'll need to add the appropriate points. If you currently stretch, weight train, or participate in a conditioning workout, finish reading this book before answering the following three questions. If you aren't doing any of the above activities, go ahead and answer questions A, B, and C.

A. Do you participate in a regular full-body weight-training workout two to three times a week?

Yes	No
5	10

Points 0

B. Do you participate in a regular full-body stretching routine four to five times a week?

Yes	No
5	10

Points 0

C. Do you participate in a regular conditioning workout at least three times a week for about 20-30 minutes?

Yes	No
5	10

Points 0

4. Do you always wear a seat belt while in a motor vehicle?

Yes	No
0	5

Points 0

5. Are you tall?

Men:

5'10" - 6'0"	over 6'0" - 6'2"
1 pt.	2 pts.
over 6'2" - 6'4"	over 6'4"
3 pts.	4 pts.

Points 0

Women:

5'5" - 5'7"	over 5'7" - 5'9"
1 pt.	2 pts.
over 5'9" - 5'11"	over 5'11"
3 pts.	4 pts.

Points 2

6. Body frame size

Women:

Small	Medium	Large
less than 5 1/4″	5 1/4-6″	more than 6″

Men:

Small	Medium	Large
less than 6 1/4″	6 1/4-7″	more than 7″

Overweight by

< 10 %	10-19%	20-29%	30-39 %	40 % or >
1 pt.	2 pts.	3 pts.	4 pts.	5 pts.

Points 0

TABLE 4-2

RISK FOR LIFTING AND CARRYING AT HOME

TIME

	1 hour or less	Occasional 1-2 hours	Intermittent 2-4 hours	Frequent 4-6 hours	Constant 6-8 hours
5-10% Minimal	1	1.5	2	3	3.5
11-25% Light	1.5	2	2-3	3-4	4-5
26-50% Moderate	2	2-3	4-5	4-6	5-7
51-75% Heavy	3	3-4	4-6	7-10	10-15
76% & up Very Heavy	3.5	4-5	5-7	10-15	20-30
Points	6.5		2		

Total Points 8.5

TABLE 4-3

MOVEMENTS DURING NONWORK ACTIVITIES

(Cross off the appropriate point box)

	Number of hours per day							
Activity	**1 hr.**	**2 hrs.**	**3 hrs.**	**4 hrs.**	**5 hrs.**	**6 hrs.**	**7 hrs.**	**8 hrs.**
Twisting	3	4	5	6	7	8	9	10
Bending forward	2	3	4	5	6	7	8	9
Reaching outward	2	3	4	5	6	7	8	9
Bending backward	1	2	3	4	5	6	7	8
Sitting	1	2	3	4	5	6	7	8
Driving	1	2	3	4	5	6	7	8
One-sided movements	1	2	3	4	5	6	7	8
Pushing & pulling	0	0	1	2	3	4	5	6
Standing	0	0	0	0	0	1	2	3
Average Daily Points	6	2						

* Driving includes, noncommute driving of cars, trucks, or recreational vehicles.

Total Points 8

DETERMINING ADDITIONAL RISK FOR WOMEN

A. Are you a Causcasian woman?

Yes	No
1	0

B. As a child and a young adult, did (do) you have a diet low in dairy products (milk, cheese, etc.)?

Yes	No
1	0

C. Do you consume a high-protein diet? Food consists of carbohydrates, protein, and fats. If you consume above 15% of your total food intake from protein, the answer is yes. Protein is found in meats, fish, beans, nuts, and dairy products.

Yes	No
1	0

D. Do you consume large amounts of caffeine (more than 4 cups of coffee, tea or cola beverages per day)?

Yes	No
1	0

Total Osteoporosis Points 1

2. Multiple pregnancies:
Number of Pregnancies

2	3	4	above 5
1	2	4	5

Total Points 4

Your total individual risk: points 43.5

OCCUPATIONAL RISK FACTORS

TABLE 4-4

RISK FOR LIFTING AND CARRYING AT WORK

TIME

	1 hour or less	Occasional 1-2 hours	Intermittent 2-4 hours	Frequent 4-6 hours	Constant 6-8 hours
5-10% Minimal	1	1.5	2	3	3.5
11-25% Light	1.5	2	2-3	3-4	4-5
26-50% Moderate	2	2-3	4-5	4-6	5-7
51-75% Heavy	3	3-4	4-6	7-10	10-15
76% & up Very Heavy	3.5	4-5	5-7	10-15	20-30
Points	4.5	3.5			

Total Points 8

TABLE 4-5

MOVEMENTS AT WORK

(Cross off the appropriate point box)

Activity	1 hr.	2 hrs.	3 hrs.	4 hrs.	5 hrs.	6 hrs.	7 hrs.	8 hrs.
	Number of hours per day							
Twisting	~~3~~	4	5	6	7	8	9	10
Bending forward	~~2~~	3	4	5	6	7	8	9
Reaching outward	~~2~~	3	4	5	6	7	8	9
Bending backward	1	2	3	4	5	6	7	8
Sitting	1	2	3	4	5	6	7	8
Driving*	1	2	3	4	5	6	7	8
Vibrational forces (e.g. jackhammer)	1	2	3	4	5	6	7	8
One-sided movements	1	2	3	4	5	6	7	8
Pushing & pulling	~~0~~	0	1	2	3	4	5	6
Standing	0	0	0	0	0	1	~~2~~	3
Average Daily Points	7						2	

* Driving includes, cars, trucks, forklifts, or other moving equipment, both at work and commuting.

Total Points 9

Your total occupation risk: Points 17

RECREATIONAL RISK FACTORS

TABLE 4-6

RECREATIONAL ACTIVITIES

	Frequency				
	Minimal	Occasional	Regular		
Activity	1-3 month	1-2 a week	3-7 a week	Annual Amount	
HOCKEY	.2	.6	.8	X	=
RODEO RIDING	.2	.6	.8	X	=
FOOTBALL/ RUGBY	.2	.6	.8	X	=
GOLF	.1	.5	.6	X	=
GYMNASTICS	.1	.5	.6	X	=
BACKPACKING	.1	.4	.5	X	=
JAVELIN THROWING	.1	.4	.5	X	=
RACQUETBALL	.1	.4	.5	X	=
BOWLING	.1	.4	.5	X	=
SQUASH	.1	.4	.5	X	=
HANDBALL	.1	.4	.5	X	=
ROWING	.1	.4	.5	X	=
JOGGING	.1	.4	.5	X	=
CROSS-COUNTRY SKIING	.1	.4	.5	X	=
WRESTLING	.1	.4	.5	X	=
BASEBALL/SOFTBALL	.1	.4	.5	X	=
TENNIS	.1	.4	.5	X	=

Your total recreational risk: Points ___0___

PSYCHOLOGICAL RISK FACTORS

The following questions deal with how your behavior may play a role in the development of back pain:

1. How would you describe your ability to tolerate pain?

Normal	Above normal	Below normal
0 pts	-3 pts	+3 pts

Points 0

2. Do you have a high level of emotional stress at home or at work?

Yes	No
+3 pts	0 pts

Points 0

3. Do you experience anxiety frequently at work or while at home?

Yes	No
+3 pts	0 pts

Points 0

Your total psychological risk: Points 0

Use the following chart to total your points in each risk category.

Your Total Points

Individual risk total	43.5
Occupational risk total	17
Recreational risk total	0
Psychological risk total	0
Total Points	60.5

Guidelines for Back Pain

Some risk	Moderate risk	High risk
< 50 pts.	50-100 pts.	> 100 pts.

Otis Before Back Building

INDIVIDUAL RISK FACTORS

1. Age

35-55	56 & up	18-34
20	15	5

Points 20

2. Smoking
Cigarettes per Day

1-5	6-10	11-20	21 or more
5	10	20	30

Points 30

3. Exercise

If you already participate in the back-friendly workout, no points will be added to the next three questions. However, if you don't participate in this workout program, you'll need to add the appropriate points. If you currently stretch, weight train, or participate in a conditioning workout, finish reading this book before answering the following three questions. If you aren't doing any of the above activities, go ahead and answer questions A, B, and C.

A. Do you participate in a regular full-body weight-training workout two to three times a week?

Yes	No
5	10

Points 10

B. Do you participate in a regular full-body stretching routine four to five times a week?

Yes	No
5	10

Points 10

C. Do you participate in a regular conditioning workout at least three times a week for about 20-30 minutes?

Yes	No
5	10

Points 10

4. Do you always wear a seat belt while in a motor vehicle?

Yes	No
0	5

Points 5

5. Are you tall?

Men:

5′10″- 6′0″	over 6′0″- 6′2″
1 pt.	2 pts.
over 6′2″- 6′4″	over 6′4″
3 pts.	4 pts.

Points 0

Women:

5′5″- 5′7″	over 5′7″- 5′9″
1 pt.	2 pts.
over 5′9″- 5′11″	over 5′11″
3 pts.	4 pts.

Points 0

6. Body frame size

   Women:

Small	Medium	Large
less than 5 1/4″	5 1/4-6″	more than 6″

   Men:

Small	Medium	Large
less than 6 1/4″	6 1/4-7″	more than 7″

   Overweight by

< 10 %	10-19%	20-29%	30-39 %	40 % or >
1 pt.	2 pts.	3 pts.	4 pts.	5 pts.

   Points 2

TABLE 4-2

RISK FOR LIFTING AND CARRYING AT HOME

TIME

	1 hour or less	Occasional 1-2 hours	Intermittent 2-4 hours	Frequent 4-6 hours	Constant 6-8 hours
5-10% Minimal	~~1~~	1.5	2	3	3.5
11-25% Light	~~1.5~~	2	2-3	3-4	4-5
26-50% Moderate	2	2-3	4-5	4-6	5-7
51-75% Heavy	3	3-4	4-6	7-10	10-15
76% & up Very Heavy	3.5	4-5	5-7	10-15	20-30
Points	2.5				

Total Points 2.5

TABLE 4-3

MOVEMENTS DURING NONWORK ACTIVITIES

(Cross off the appropriate point box)

	Number of hours per day							
Activity	**1 hr.**	**2 hrs.**	**3 hrs.**	**4 hrs.**	**5 hrs.**	**6 hrs.**	**7 hrs.**	**8 hrs.**
Twisting	3	4	5	6	7	8	9	10
Bending forward	2	3	4	5	6	7	8	9
Reaching outward	2	3	4	5	6	7	8	9
Bending backward	1	2	3	4	5	6	7	8
Sitting	1	2	3	4	5	6	7	8
Driving	~~1~~	2	3	4	5	6	7	8
One-sided movements	~~1~~	2	3	4	5	6	7	8
Pushing & pulling	0	0	1	2	3	4	5	6
Standing	0	0	0	0	0	1	2	3
Average Daily Points	2							

* Driving includes, noncommute driving of cars, trucks, or recreational vehicles.

Total Points 2

DETERMINING ADDITIONAL RISK FOR WOMEN

A. Are you a Causcasian woman?

Yes	No
1	0

B. As a child and a young adult, did (do) you have a diet low in dairy products (milk, cheese, etc.)?

Yes	No
1	0

C. Do you consume a high-protein diet? Food consists of carbohydrates, protein, and fats. If you consume above 15% of your total food intake from protein, the answer is yes. Protein is found in meats, fish, beans, nuts, and dairy products.

Yes	No
1	0

D. Do you consume large amounts of caffeine (more than 4 cups of coffee, tea or cola beverages per day)?

Yes	No
1	0

Total Osteoporosis Points __________

2. Multiple pregnancies:
Number of Pregnancies

2	3	4	above 5
1	2	4	5

Total Points 0

Your total individual risk: points 91.5

OCCUPATIONAL RISK FACTORS

TABLE 4-4

RISK FOR LIFTING AND CARRYING AT WORK

TIME

	1 hour or less	Occasional 1-2 hours	Intermittent 2-4 hours	Frequent 4-6 hours	Constant 6-8 hours
5-10% Minimal	1	1.5	2	3	3.5
11-25% Light	1.5	2	2-3	3-4	4-5
26-50% Moderate	2	2-3	4-5	4-6	5-7
51-75% Heavy	3	3-4	4-6	7-10	10-15
76% & up Very Heavy	3.5	4-5	5-7	10-15	20-30
Points	1				

Total Points 1

TABLE 4-5

MOVEMENTS AT WORK

(Cross off the appropriate point box)

Activity	Number of hours per day 1 hr.	2 hrs.	3 hrs.	4 hrs.	5 hrs.	6 hrs.	7 hrs.	8 hrs.
Twisting	3	4	5	6	7	8	9	10
Bending forward	~~2~~	3	4	5	6	7	8	9
Reaching outward	2	3	4	5	6	7	8	9
Bending backward	1	2	3	4	5	6	7	8
Sitting	1	2	3	4	5	~~6~~	7	8
Driving*	1	2	~~3~~	4	5	6	7	8
Vibrational forces (e.g. jackhammer)	1	2	3	4	5	6	7	8
One-sided movements	~~1~~	2	3	4	5	6	7	8
Pushing & pulling	0	0	1	2	3	4	5	6
Standing	0	0	0	0	0	1	2	3
Average Daily Points	3		3			6		

* Driving includes, cars, trucks, forklifts, or other moving equipment, both at work and commuting.

Total Points 12

Your total occupation risk: Points 13

RECREATIONAL RISK FACTORS

TABLE 4-6
RECREATIONAL ACTIVITIES

	Frequency				
	Minimal	Occasional	Regular		
Activity	1-3 month	1-2 a week	3-7 a week	Annual Amount	
HOCKEY	.2	.6	.8	X	=
RODEO RIDING	.2	.6	.8	X	=
FOOTBALL/ RUGBY	.2	.6	.8	X	=
GOLF	.1	.5	.6	X 47	= 28.2
GYMNASTICS	.1	.5	.6	X	=
BACKPACKING	.1	.4	.5	X	=
JAVELIN THROWING	.1	.4	.5	X	=
RACQUETBALL	.1	.4	.5	X	=
BOWLING	.1	.4	.5	X	=
SQUASH	.1	.4	.5	X	=
HANDBALL	.1	.4	.5	X	=
ROWING	.1	.4	.5	X	=
JOGGING	.1	.4	.5	X	=
CROSS-COUNTRY SKIING	.1	.4	.5	X	=
WRESTLING	.1	.4	.5	X	=
BASEBALL/SOFTBALL	.1	.4	.5	X	=
TENNIS	.1	.4	.5	X	=

Your total recreational risk: Points 28.2

PSYCHOLOGICAL RISK FACTORS

The following questions deal with how your behavior may play a role in the development of back pain:

1. How would you describe your ability to tolerate pain?

Normal	Above normal	Below normal
0 pts	-3 pts	+3 pts

Points 3

2. Do you have a high level of emotional stress at home or at work?

Yes	No
+3 pts	0 pts

Points 3

3. Do you experience anxiety frequently at work or while at home?

Yes	No
+3 pts	0 pts

Points 3

Your total psychological risk: Points 9

Use the following chart to total your points in each risk category.

Your Total Points

Individual risk total	91.5
Occupational risk total	13
Recreational risk total	28.2
Psychological risk total	9
Total Points	141.7

Guidelines for Back Pain

Some risk	Moderate risk	High risk
< 50 pts.	50-100 pts.	> 100 pts.

Otis After Back Building

INDIVIDUAL RISK FACTORS

1. Age

35-55	56 & up	18-34
20	15	5

Points 20

2. Smoking
Cigarettes per Day

1-5	6-10	11-20	21 or more
5	10	20	30

Points 0

3. Exercise

If you already participate in the back-friendly workout, no points will be added to the next three questions. However, if you don't participate in this workout program, you'll need to add the appropriate points. If you currently stretch, weight train, or participate in a conditioning workout, finish reading this book before answering the following three questions. If you aren't doing any of the above activities, go ahead and answer questions A, B, and C.

A. Do you participate in a regular full-body weight-training workout two to three times a week?

Yes	No
5	10

Points 0

B. Do you participate in a regular full-body stretching routine four to five times a week?

Yes	No
5	10

Points 0

C. Do you participate in a regular conditioning workout at least three times a week for about 20-30 minutes?

Yes	No
5	10

Points 0

4. Do you always wear a seat belt while in a motor vehicle?

Yes	No
0	5

Points 0

5. Are you tall?

Men:

5′10″- 6′0″	over 6′0″- 6′2″
1 pt.	2 pts.
over 6′2″- 6′4″	over 6′4″
3 pts.	4 pts.

Points 0

Women:

5′5″- 5′7″	over 5′7″- 5′9″
1 pt.	2 pts.
over 5′9″- 5′11″	over 5′11″
3 pts.	4 pts.

Points 0

6. Body frame size

Women:

Small	Medium	Large
less than 5 1/4"	5 1/4-6"	more than 6"

Men:

Small	Medium	Large
less than 6 1/4"	6 1/4-7"	more than 7"

Overweight by

≤ 10 %	10-19%	20-29%	30-39 %	40 % or ≥
1 pt.	2 pts.	3 pts.	4 pts.	5 pts.

Points 0

TABLE 4-2

RISK FOR LIFTING AND CARRYING AT HOME

TIME

	1 hour or less	Occasional 1-2 hours	Intermittent 2-4 hours	Frequent 4-6 hours	Constant 6-8 hours
5-10% Minimal	~~1~~	1.5	2	3	3.5
11-25% Light	1.5	2	2-3	3-4	4-5
26-50% Moderate	2	2-3	4-5	4-6	5-7
51-75% Heavy	3	3-4	4-6	7-10	10-15
76% & up Very Heavy	3.5	4-5	5-7	10-15	20-30
Points	1				

Total Points 1

TABLE 4-3

MOVEMENTS DURING NONWORK ACTIVITIES

(Cross off the appropriate point box)

Activity	Number of hours per day 1 hr.	2 hrs.	3 hrs.	4 hrs.	5 hrs.	6 hrs.	7 hrs.	8 hrs.
Twisting	3	4	5	6	7	8	9	10
Bending forward	2	3	4	5	6	7	8	9
Reaching outward	2	3	4	5	6	7	8	9
Bending backward	1	2	3	4	5	6	7	8
Sitting	1	2	3	4	5	6	7	8
Driving	~~1~~	2	3	4	5	6	7	8
One-sided movements	1	2	3	4	5	6	7	8
Pushing & pulling	0	0	1	2	3	4	5	6
Standing	0	0	0	0	0	1	2	3
Average Daily Points	1							

* Driving includes, noncommute driving of cars, trucks, or recreational vehicles.

Total Points 1

DETERMINING ADDITIONAL RISK FOR WOMEN

A. Are you a Causcasian woman?

Yes	No
1	0

B. As a child and a young adult, did (do) you have a diet low in dairy products (milk, cheese, etc.)?

Yes	No
1	0

C. Do you consume a high-protein diet? Food consists of carbohydrates, protein, and fats. If you consume above 15% of your total food intake from protein, the answer is yes. Protein is found in meats, fish, beans, nuts, and dairy products.

Yes	No
1	0

D. Do you consume large amounts of caffeine (more than 4 cups of coffee, tea or cola beverages per day)?

Yes	No
1	0

Total Osteoporosis Points ____0____

2. Multiple pregnancies:
Number of Pregnancies

2	3	4	above 5
1	2	4	5

Total Points ____0____

Your total individual risk: points ____22____

OCCUPATIONAL RISK FACTORS

TABLE 4-4

RISK FOR LIFTING AND CARRYING AT WORK

TIME

	1 hour or less	Occasional 1-2 hours	Intermittent 2-4 hours	Frequent 4-6 hours	Constant 6-8 hours
5-10% Minimal	1	1.5	2	3	3.5
11-25% Light	1.5	2	2-3	3-4	4-5
26-50% Moderate	2	2-3	4-5	4-6	5-7
51-75% Heavy	3	3-4	4-6	7-10	10-15
76% & up Very Heavy	3.5	4-5	5-7	10-15	20-30

Points	1				

Total Points 1

TABLE 4-5
MOVEMENTS AT WORK

(Cross off the appropriate point box)

Activity	1 hr.	2 hrs.	3 hrs.	4 hrs.	5 hrs.	6 hrs.	7 hrs.	8 hrs.
	Number of hours per day							
Twisting	3	4	5	6	7	8	9	10
Bending forward	~~2~~	3	4	5	6	7	8	9
Reaching outward	2	3	4	5	6	7	8	9
Bending backward	1	2	3	4	5	6	7	8
Sitting	1	2	3	4	~~5~~	6	7	8
Driving*	1	2	~~3~~	4	5	6	7	8
Vibrational forces (e.g. jackhammer)	1	2	3	4	5	6	7	8
One-sided movements	~~1~~	2	3	4	5	6	7	8
Pushing & pulling	0	0	1	2	3	4	5	6
Standing	0	0	0	0	0	1	2	3
Average Daily Points	3		3		5			

* Driving includes, cars, trucks, forklifts, or other moving equipment, both at work and commuting.

Total Points 11

Your total occupation risk: Points 12

RECREATIONAL RISK FACTORS

TABLE 4-6

RECREATIONAL ACTIVITIES

	Frequency				
	Minimal	Occasional	Regular		
Activity	1-3 month	1-2 a week	3-7 a week	Annual Amount	
HOCKEY	.2	.6	.8	X	=
RODEO RIDING	.2	.6	.8	X	=
FOOTBALL/ RUGBY	.2	.6	.8	X	=
GOLF	.1	.5	.6	X	=
GYMNASTICS	.1	.5	.6	X	=
BACKPACKING	.1	.4	.5	X	=
JAVELIN THROWING	.1	.4	.5	X	=
RACQUETBALL	.1	.4	.5	X	=
BOWLING	.1	.4	.5	X	=
SQUASH	.1	.4	.5	X	=
HANDBALL	.1	.4	.5	X	=
ROWING	.1	.4	.5	X	=
JOGGING	.1	.4	.5	X	=
CROSS-COUNTRY SKIING	.1	.4	.5	X	=
WRESTLING	.1	.4	.5	X	=
BASEBALL/SOFTBALL	.1	.4	.5	X	=
TENNIS	.1	.4	.5	X	=

Your total recreational risk: Points ___0___

PSYCHOLOGICAL RISK FACTORS

The following questions deal with how your behavior may play a role in the development of back pain:

1. How would you describe your ability to tolerate pain?

Normal	Above normal	Below normal
0 pts	-3 pts	+3 pts

Points 0

2. Do you have a high level of emotional stress at home or at work?

Yes	No
+3 pts	0 pts

Points 0

3. Do you experience anxiety frequently at work or while at home?

Yes	No
+3 pts	0 pts

Points 0

Your total psychological risk: Points 0

Use the following chart to total your points in each risk category.

Your Total Points

Individual risk total	22
Occupational risk total	12
Recreational risk total	0
Psychological risk total	0
Total Points	34

Guidelines for Back Pain

Some risk	Moderate risk	High risk
< 50 pts.	50-100 pts.	> 100 pts.

APPENDIX D

MATERIALS FOR STAYING MOTIVATED

The Back-Friendly Workout Personal Exercise Contract

I, ______________________ am contracting with myself to agree to participate in the back-friendly workout. I agree that I will choose to participate in a complete exercise program that will include a warm-up and cool-down, weight training, and conditioning. I also agree to maintain a daily workout log of my activity. I will plan to set aside an unconditional part of my daily or weekly schedule to exercise. In addition, I will assess my workout log periodically to determine whether I am reaching or maintaining my desired goals. If not, I will agree to find ways to accomplish such goals.

Signed __________________ Date _________

Witness _________________

Back-Friendly Workout

ANNUAL POINT SYSTEM

To encourage you to partipate in a complete exercise routine, record points for each type of exercise you performed. In addition, you're awarded a bonus of six points if you accomplish three conditioning workouts , two upper and lower body weight-training workouts, and seven warm-up exercises in one week. This will give you a possible total of twenty points per week.

Week	Points
1	
2	
3	
4	
5	
6	
7	
8	
9	
10	
11	
12	
13	
14	
15	
16	
17	
18	
19	
20	
21	
22	
23	
24	
25	
26	

Week	Points
27	
28	
29	
30	
31	
32	
33	
34	
35	
36	
37	
38	
39	
40	
41	
42	
43	
44	
45	
46	
47	
48	
49	
50	
51	
52	

(27-51) Subtotal ________

(1-26) Subtotal ________

Total ________

Back-Friendly Workout Conditioning Log

NAME ______________________________

Week	Day	Type of Conditioning	Heart Rate Training Level	Borgs Scale (6-20)	Duration

Back-Friendly Workout Warm-up Exercise Log

NAME ______________________________

Week	Day	Mid-back	Back of Thigh	Buttocks	Back	Front Thigh	Hip Flexors	Calf	Inner Thigh	Outer Thigh & Hip	Back & Ribcage	Upper Back & Front Arms	Upper Back, Arms, Shoulders	Chest	Shoulders	Neck

Back-Friendly Workout Cool-Down Exercise Log

NAME ______________________

Week	Day	Back of Thigh	Back	Hip Flexor	Back & Ribcage	Chest	Neck

Back-Friendly Workout Weight-Training Log

NAME ______________________________

			Lower Body									Upper Body							
Week	Day	Sets Repetitions	Back Extensions	Knee Extensors	Lunges	Toe Raises	Leg Push	Leg Pulls	Knee Raises	Leg Curls		Shoulder Shrugs	Pull-downs	Neck	Push-downs	Overhead Press	Incline Bench Press	Bench Press	Curls
		2 3																	
		8 10 12																	
		2 3																	
		8 10 12																	
		2 3																	
		8 10 12																	
		2 3																	
		8 10 12																	
		2 3																	
		8 10 12																	
		2 3																	
		8 10 12																	
		2 3																	
		8 10 12																	
		2 3																	
		8 10 12																	
		2 3																	
		8 10 12																	
		2 3																	
		8 10 12																	
		2 3																	
		8 10 12																	
		2 3																	
		8 10 12																	

Appendix E

EXERCISES TO AVOID

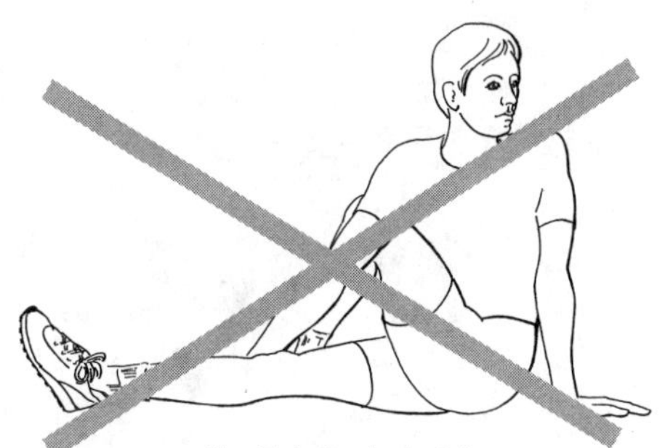

Fig. E-1. Body twist

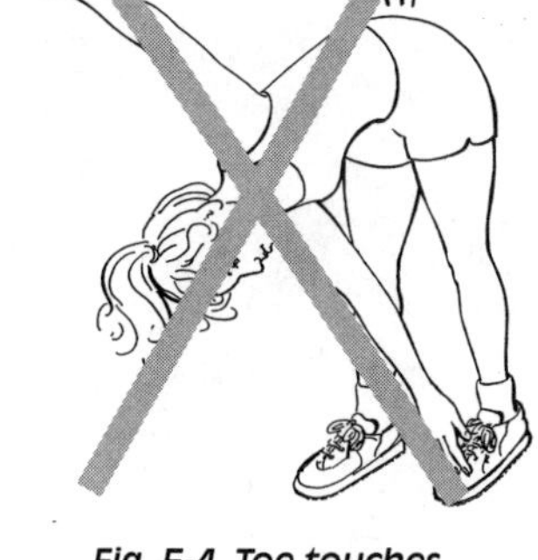

Fig. E-4. Toe touches

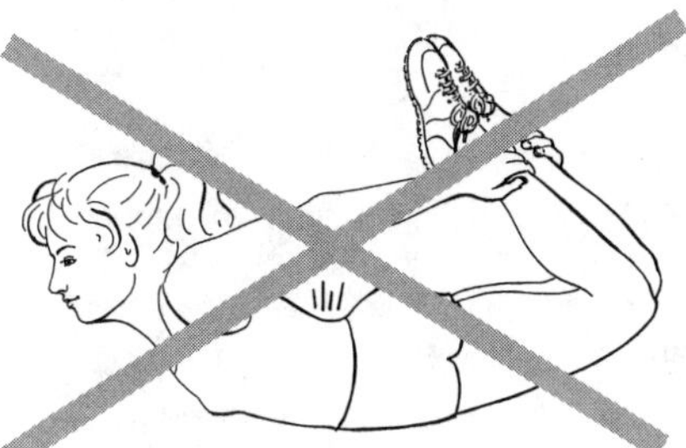

Fig. E-2. Arching back

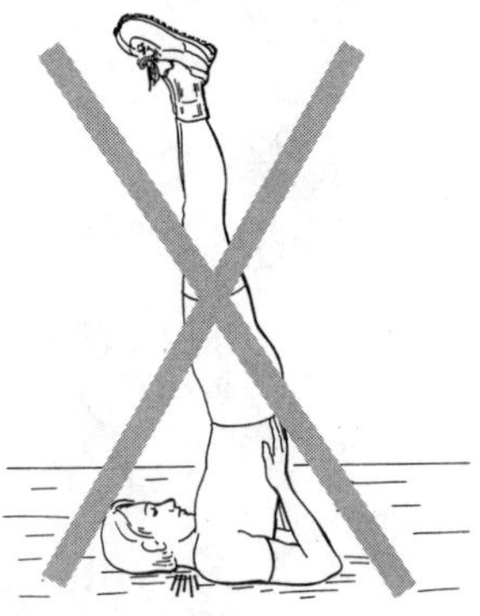

Fig. E-5. Shoulder stand

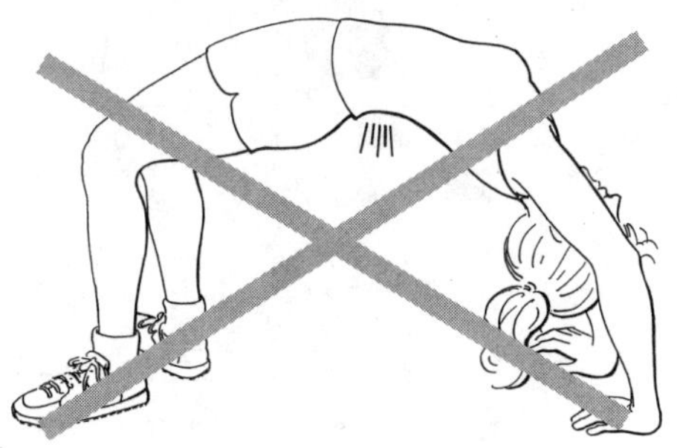

Fig. E-3. Upward body lift

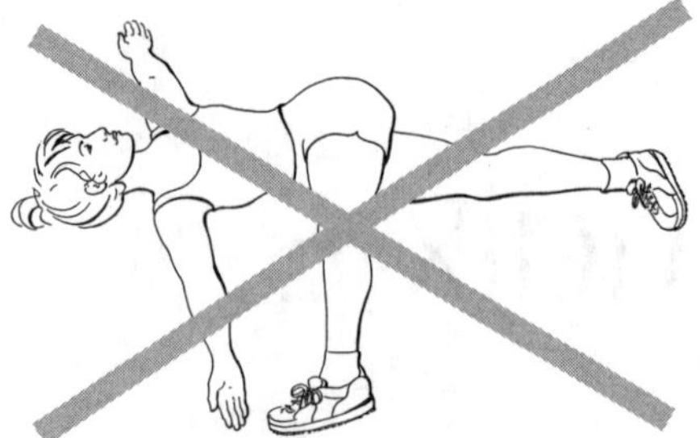

Fig. E-6. Leg twist

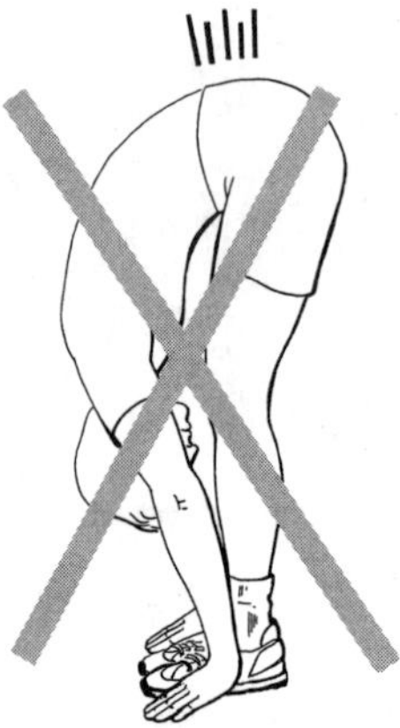

Fig. E-7. Hands to floor

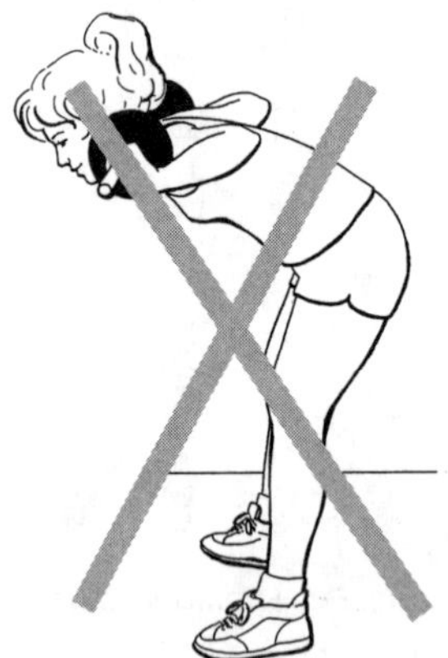

Fig. E-8. Good morning stretch

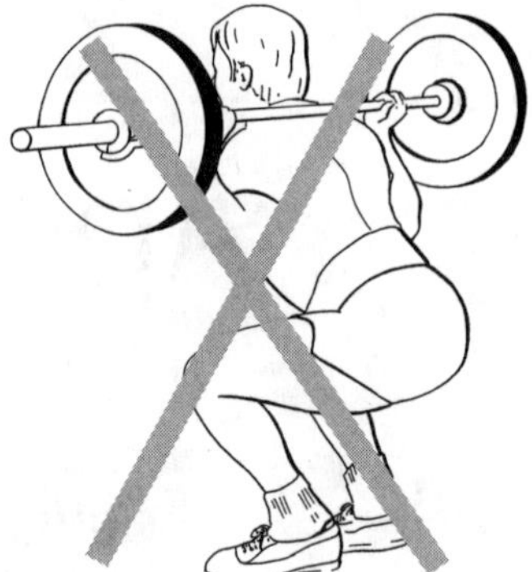

Fig. E-9. Squats

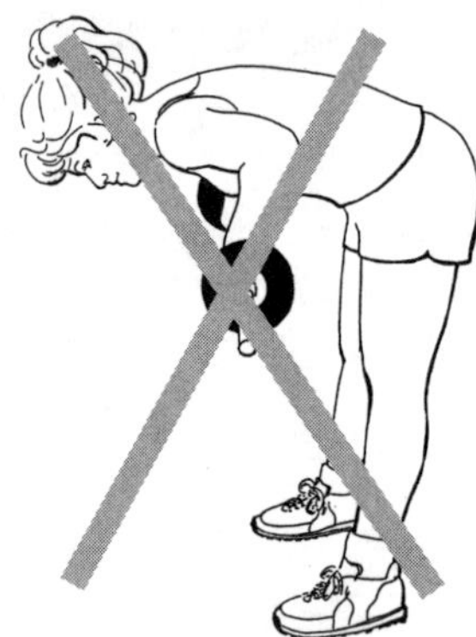

Fig. E-10. Bent-over rows

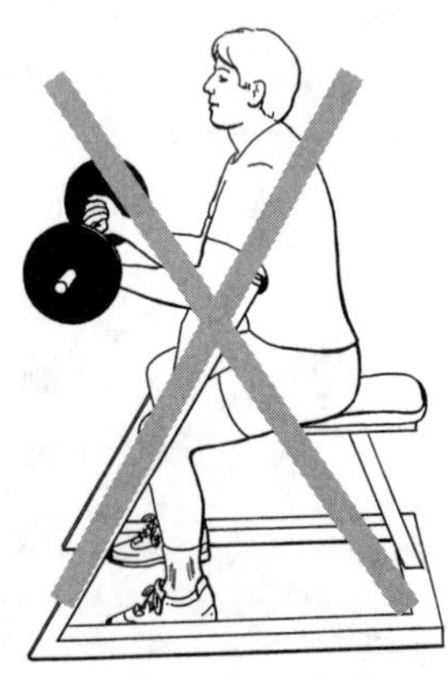

Fig. E-11. Preacher curls

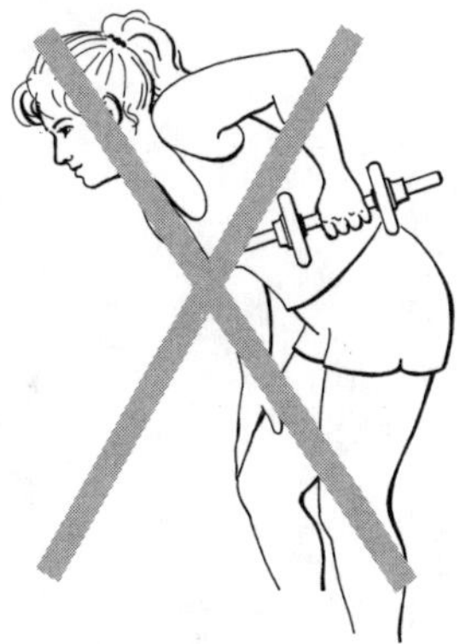

Fig. E-12. Dumbbell bent-over rows

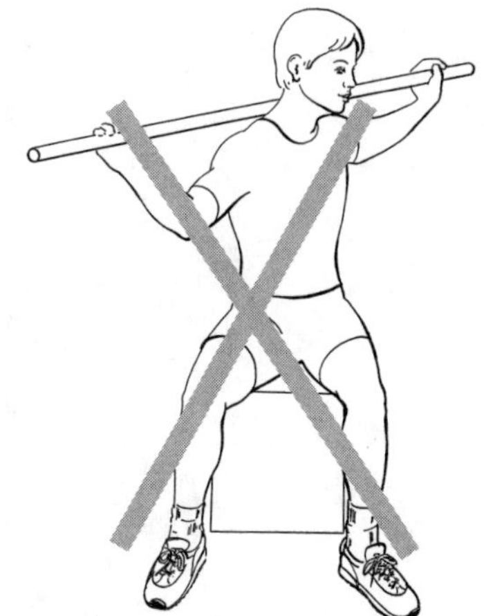

Fig. E-15. Bar twists

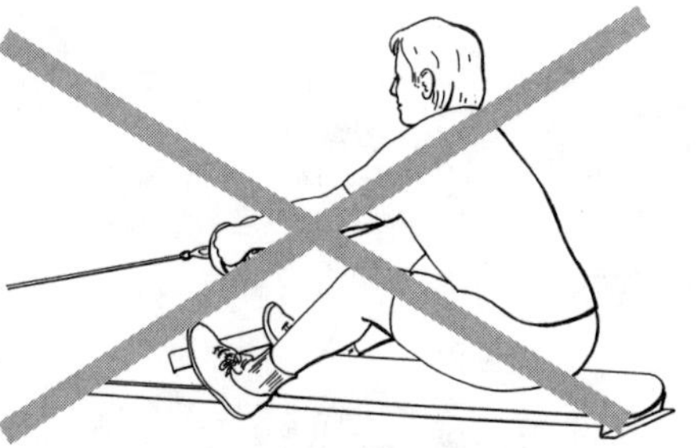

Fig. E-13. Seated rows

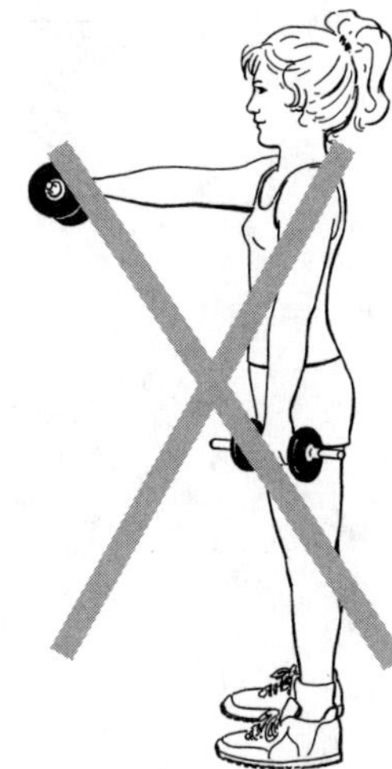

Fig. E-16. Front raises

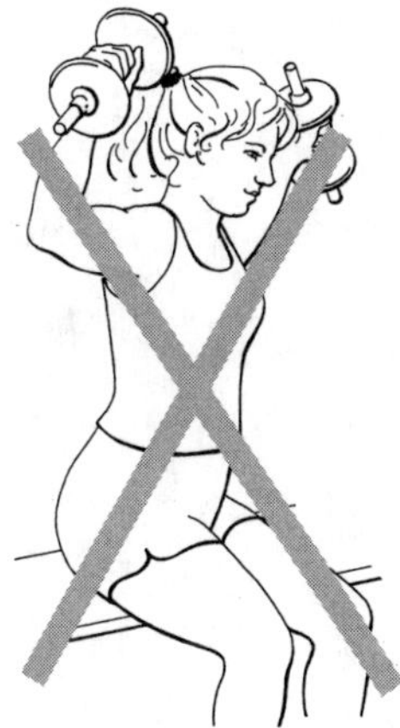

Fig. E-14. Fly's

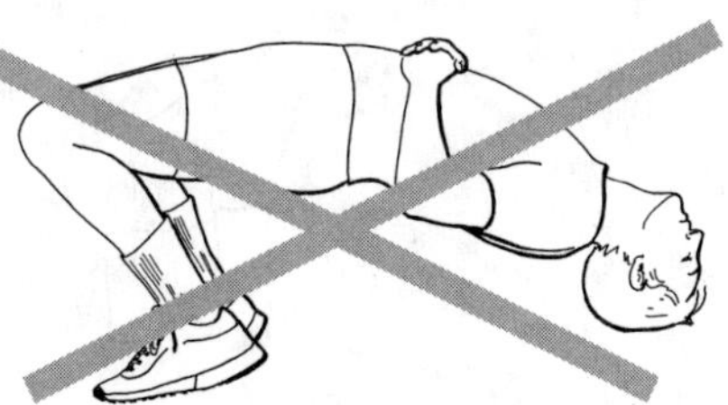

Fig. E-17. Neck bridges

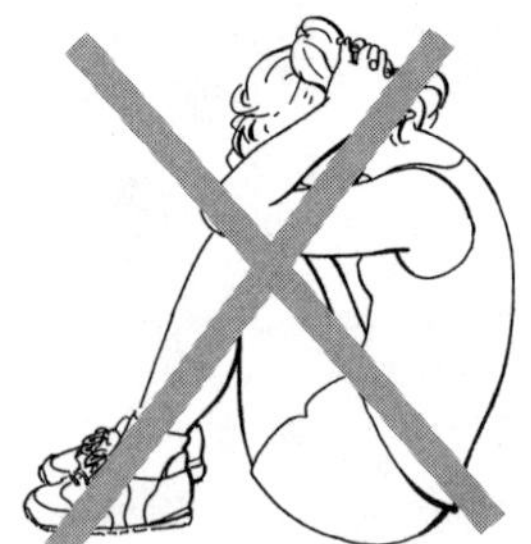

Fig. E-18. Sit-ups

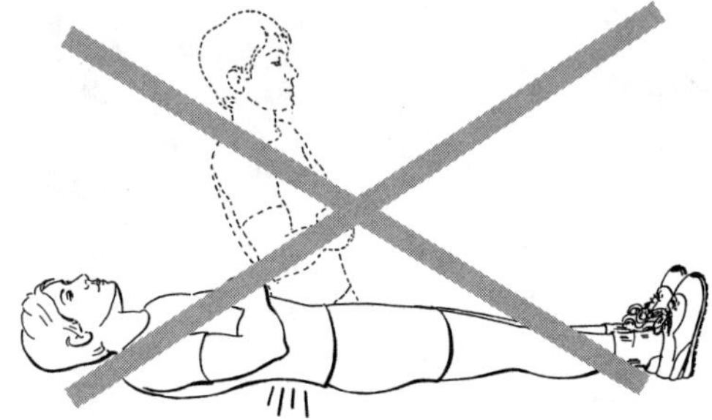

Fig. E-19. Back lifts

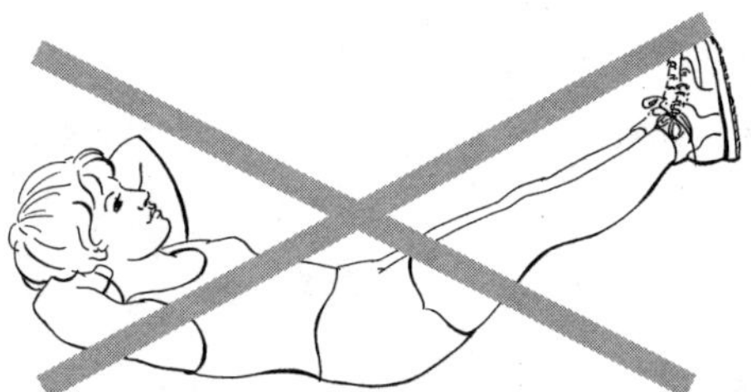

Fig. E-20. Leg lifts

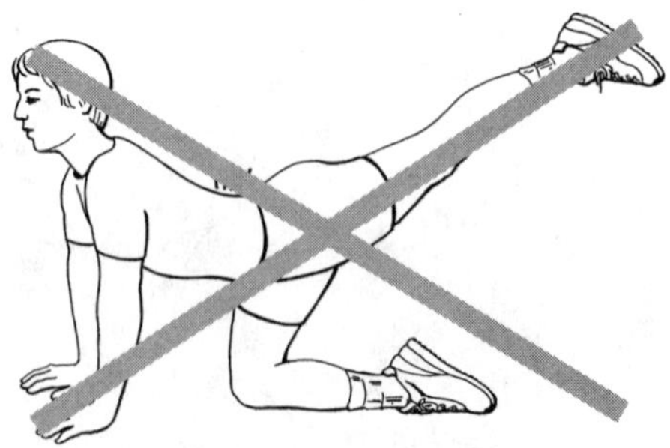

Fig. E-21. Backward leg kicks

Back-Building Terms

Advancing age: An individual risk factor for back pain. The older you get and the more risk factors you're exposed to during your lifetime, the likelihood of developing back pain increases.

Back school: An educational program that gives you practical advice on how to prevent back pain and control it once it has developed. This is usually done through demonstrating proper body mechanics for common daily activities and teaching self-help procedures if pain does occur.

Body composition: The percentage of body fat compared to lean body mass (muscle, bone, and vital organs). Having the proper body composition is a component of being physically fit.

Cardiovascular conditioning: Exercise in which your heart and lungs work harder to supply adequate oxygen to the body for long periods of time.

Disc: Located between the vertebrae in the spinal column, a disc acts as a shock absorber and allows flexibility within the spine (refer to Fig. 2-4).

Duration: The amount of time spent exercising.

Endorphins: Natural chemical releases within the nervous system that relieve pain.

Ergonomics: The science of proper mechanical use of the human body within its environment. Ergonomics is mostly studied within the workplace or applied to equipment used in the workplace.

Extrinsic motivation: A person who seeks motivation from an outside source, such as receiving a trophy, money, praise, or public recognition. An exercise contract, log, and a point system have been developed to keep you motivated (see Appendix D).

Flexibility: The ability of a joint or muscle to move within its full range of motion.

Frequency: How often a person exercises.

Health conditions: Many conditions and diseases, some of which are not preventable, can cause back pain (refer to Table 3-2).

Herniated disc: Displacement of the inner core beyond the outer boundary of the disc.

Illness behavior: Occurs when perceived pain and disability are greater than the actual level of pain and disability. People with back pain who have been inactive for a prolonged period tend to develop a fear of pain, keeping them further inactive or disabled. People without this behavior are those who work or remain active after a similar injury. In addition, an illness behavior can develop if disability is present and legal and economic factors influence a person's perceived pain level.

Inner core: The jellylike center of a disc is mainly made of water (refer to fig 2-5). This part of the disc allows the spine to have a shock-absorbing ability.

Intensity: The level of difficultly of an exercise session.

Intrinsic motivation: Motivation found from within a person. People who love to participate in a certain recreational activity create an inner satisfaction that keeps them motivated. In addition, those who spend a lot of time at something tend to become good at what they do. This can create a sense of competence, which can further keep a person motivated. Such types of rewards tend to be long lasting.

Ligament: A tough yet elastic tissue that connects bones and supports joints within the body (refer to Fig. 2-8).

Muscle endurance: The amount of time muscles can exert a force without tiring.

Muscle strength: The amount of force produced by muscle groups as evidenced by how much weight you can lift.

Multiple pregnancies: For every increase in pregnancy and delivery a woman endures, the greater the risk of back pain.

Nerve roots: Cordlike structures of nerve fibers that leave the spinal cord and branch throughout the body, passing through the spinal column near the joints and discs of the moveable vertebrae (refer to Fig. 2-9). The sacrum and tailbone have openings on both sides where the nerve roots pass.

Osteoporosis: Thinning of the bones, commonly found among elderly women. Symptoms develop when bones become so weak that they collapse or break. Osteoporosis in the spine can lead to a permanent hump in the back (refer to Fig. 3-1b).

Outer boundary: A tough, fibrous band located on the outside of a disc (refer to Fig. 2-5). This outer boundary is susceptible to damage as a result of a person's lifestyle.

Pain behavior: The behavioral response to the stimulus and tolerance of pain. The higher the pain tolerance, the less likely one is to feel pain.

Postural deformities: Structural changes, often the result of birth, of the bones and joints that affect the spine. Such changes include the normal curves of the spine and unequal leg length.

Primary prevention approach: A method of preventing certain health conditions before they develop.

Repetition: One complete cycle of a weight-training exercise (such as raising the bar upward in bench press, then lowering it)

Sacrum: A bone structure of fused vertebrae located within the spinal column below the low-back vertebrae and between the two hip bones (refer to Fig. 2-3)

Set: A group of 8-12 repetitions performed without resting during weight training. Normally, 2-3 sets are performed for each exercise.

Smoking: The act of inhaling tobacco. This is a risk factor for back pain because it lowers the amount of oxygen needed to maintain a healthy spine.

Spinal column: A series of joined vertebrae forming the central support of the skeleton, commonly called the backbone (refer to Fig. 2-1).

Spinal cord: Part of the central nervous system that extends down from the brain within the spinal column.

Spondylolisthesis: Similar to a spondylolysis, except there is a forward displacement of the front part of a vertebra over the segment below. Usually found in the lowest two vertebrae in the low back (refer to Fig. 3- 4b). This condition can be painless and therefore often remains undetected.

Spondylolysis: This condition has a separation of the bony structures within the middle section of a vertebra and is usually present in the low back. No forward displacement of the front part of the vertebra is present. There are a number of causes for this condition: (1) as a result of a possible birth defect, cartilage is present in adulthood instead of bone; (2) separation of a vertebra occurs as a result of trauma, such as a football or gymnastics injury; (3) degeneration and erosion of a vertebra among the elderly can cause the vertebra to break.

Spotter: A weight-training helper to ensure safety to the lifter

Steroids: Hormones used to enhance muscle size and strength. Often sold illegally and should be avoided (refer to Table 10-3).

Tailbone: The lowest bony structure found within the spinal column (refer to Fig. 2-3).

Target heart rate: The heart rate desired by an individual to achieve cardiovascular conditioning (refer to Table 9-1 and Fig. 9-1 and 9-2).

Treatment approach: A method to promote health by treating a disease or health condition once it has occurred.

Vertebrae: The bony segments within the spinal column (refer to Fig. 2-3). There are 33 vertebrae in the spinal column: 7 in the neck, 12 in the mid-back, 5 in the low back, 5 in the sacrum, and 4 in the tailbone. A single bony segment within the neck, mid-back and low back is described as a vertebra.

Work hardening: A rehabilitation program using conditioning tasks (in conjunction with real or simulated work activities) that are graded to progressively improve the mechanical, muscular, cardiovascular and psychosocial function of an injured person, to maximize the ability to return to work. Work hardening is sometimes used to test the individual's ability to return to work.

Bibliography

These references are listed in the order that they were used in each chapter.

Chapter 1

1. Cypress, B.K. (1983). Characteristics of physician visits for back symptoms: A national perspective. American Journal of Public Health; 73 (4): 389-95.
2 American College of Sports Medicine (1986). Guidelines for exercise testing and prescription. Philadelphia: Lea & Febiger; p. 31.
3. Kirkaldy-Willis, W.H. (1983). Managing low back pain. New York: Churchill Livingstone; pp. 75-91.
4. White, A.H. (1983). Back school and other conservative approaches to low back pain. St. Louis: C.V. Mosby; p. 1.
5. Spengler, D.M.; et al. (1986). Back injuries in industry: a retrospective study. Part I overview and cost analysis. Spine; 11 (3): 241-5.
6. Nachemson, A.L. (1976). The lumbar spine: An orthopedic challenge; Spine; 1 (1): 59-71.
7. Tornatora, B.; et al (1994). Identification of risk components in exercise for the low back. Chiropractic Technique; 6 (3): 79-83.
8. Snook, S.H. (1987). Approaches to the control of back pain in industry: Job design, job placement and educational training. Spine; State of the Art Reviews; 2 (1): 45-59.
9. Fahrni, H.W. (1975). Conservative treatment of lumbar disc degeneration: Our primary responsibility. Orthopedic Clinics of North America; 6: 93-103.

10. Harris, S.S.; et al. (1989). Physical activity counseling for healthy adults as a primary preventive intervention in the clinical setting. Journal of the American Medical Association; 261 (24): 3590-8.

11. Paffenbarger, R.S.; et al. (1986). Physical activity, all-cause mortality, and longevity of college alumni. New England Journal of Medicine; 314 (10): 605-13.

12. Frontera, W.R.; et al. (1988). Strength conditioning in older men: Skeletal muscle hypertrophy and improved function. Journal of Applied Physiology; 64: 1038-44.

13. Dewitt, J.; Roberts, T. (1991). Pumping up an adult fitness program. Journal of Physical Education, Recreation and Dance. September; 67-71.

14. Kavanagh, T.; Shephard, R.J. (1990). Can regular sport participation slow the aging process? Data on masters athletes. The Physician and Sportsmedicine; 18 (6): 94-104.

15. Fiatarone, M.A.; et al. (1994). Exercise training and nutritional supplementation for physical frailty in very elderly people. The New England Journal of Medicine; 330 (25): 1769-75.

Chapter 2

1. Warwick, R.; Williams, P.L (1973). Gray's Anatomy, 35th British edition. Philadelphia: W.B. Saunders Co.

2. White, A. A.; Panjabi, M.M.(1978). Clinical Biomechanics of the Spine. Philadelphia: J.B. Lippincott Company; pp. 1-8, 13, 17-19, 45-51, 64.

3. Rudert, M.; Tillmann, B. (1993). Lymph and blood supply of the human intervertebral disc: Cadaver study of correlations to discitis. Acta Orhop Scand; 64: 37-40.

4. Lewit, K. (1985). Manipulative therapy in rehabilitation of the motor system. Butterworths; pp. 29-33.

5. Jensen, M.C.; et al. (1994). Magnetic resonance imaging of the lumbar spine in people without back pain. The New England Journal of Medicine; 331 (2): 69-73.

Chapter 3

1. Deyo, R.A. (1983). Conservative therapy for low back pain. Journal of the American Medical Association; 250 (8): 1057-62.
2. Deyo, R.A.; et al. (1992). Cost, controversy, crisis: Low back pain and the health of the public. Annual Review of Public Health; 12: 141-56.
3. Jensen, M.C.; et al. (1994). Magnetic resonance imaging of the lumbar spine in people without back pain. The New England Journal of Medicine; 331 (2): 69-73.
4. Hazard, R.C.; et al. (1989). Functional restoration with behavioral support: A one year prospective study of patients with chronic low-back pain. Spine; 14 (2): 157-61.
5. Frymoyer, J.W.; Mooney, V. (1986). Occupational orthopaedics. The Journal of Bone and Joint Surgery; 68-A (3): 469-74.
6. Troup, J.D.G. (1988). The perception of musculoskeletal pain and incapacity for work: Prevention and early treatment. Physiotherapy; 74 (9): 436-9.
7. Liebenson, C.S. (1992). Pathogenesis of chronic back pain. Journal of Manipulative and Physiological Therapeutics; 15 (5): 299-308.
8. Dillane, J.B. (1966). Acute back syndrome: A study from general practice. British Medical Journal; 2: 82-4.
9. Kirkaldy-Willis, W.H. (1985). Spinal manipulation in the treatment of low-back pain. Canada Family Physician 31; 535-40.
10. Andersson, G.B.J. (1992). Factors important in the genesis and prevention of occupational back pain and disability. Journal of Manipulative and Physiological Therapeutics; 15 (1): 43-6.
11. Wohl, A.R.; et al. (1995). Occupational injury in female aerospace workers. Epidemiology; 6 (2): 110-14.
12. Deyo, R.A.; et al. (1987). Lifestyle and low back pain: The influence of smoking, exercise and obesity. Clinical Research; 35 (3): 577 A.
13. Cady, L.D.; et al. (1979). Strength and fitness and subsequent back injuries in firefighters. Journal of Occupational Medicine; 21 (4): 269-72.
14. Cady, L.D.; et al. (1985). Program for increasing health and physical fitness of firefighters. Journal of Occupational Medicine; 27 (2): 110-14.
15. Battie, M.C.; et al. (1990). The role of spinal flexibility in back pain complaints within industry: A prospective study. Spine; 15 (8): 768-73.

16. Deyo, R.A.; et al. (1992). What can the history and physical examination tell us about low back pain? Journal of the American Medical Association; 268 (6): 760-5.

17. Chaffin, D.B.; et al. (1973). A longitudinal study of low back pain as associated with occupational weight-lifting factors. American Industrial Hygiene Association Journal; 34: 513-25.

18. Nachemson, A.L. (1976). The lumbar spine an orthopedic challenge. Spine; 1 (1): 59-71.

19. Frymoyer, J.W.; et al. (1983). Risk factors in low back pain. The Journal of Bone and Joint Surgery; 65-A (2): 213-18.

20. Hellsing, A.; et al. (1986). Individual predictability of back trouble in 18-year old men. Manual Medicine; 2: 72-6.

21. Snook, S.H. (1987). Approaches to the control of back pain in industry: Job design, job placement and educational training. Spine; State of the Art Reviews; 2 (1): 45-59.

22. Frymoyer, J.W. (1984). Helping your patients avoid low back pain. The Journal of Musculoskeletal Medicine; 1 (3): 65-74.

23. Kelsey, J.L.; et al. (1975). Driving of motor vehicles as a risk factor for acute herniated lumbar intervertebral disc. American Journal of Epidemiology; 102: 63.

24. Tewes, D.P.; et al. (1995). Lumbar transverse process fractures in professional football players. The American Journal of Sports Medicine; 23 (4): 507-9.

25. Silver, J.R. (1992). Injuries of the spine sustained during rugby. British Journal of Sports Medicine; 26 (4): 253-8.

26. Scher, A.T. (1990). Premature onset of degenerative disease of the cervical spine in rugby players. South African Medical Journal; 77 (11): 557-8.

27. Nebergall, R.W.; et al. (1992). Rough riders. The Physician and Sportsmedicine; 20 (10): 85-92.

28. Griffin, R.; et al. (1987) Injuries in professional rodeo: An update. The Physician and Sportsmedicine; 15 (2): 104-15.

29. Meyers, M.C.; et al. (1990). Injuries in intercollegiate rodeo athletes. American Journal of Sports Medicine; 18 (1): 87-91.

30. Mackie, S.J.; Taunton, J.E. (1994). Injuries in female gymnasts. The Physician and Sportsmedicine; 22 (8): 40-5.

31. Reynen, P.D.; Clancy, W.G. (1994). Cervical spine injury, hockey helmets, and face masks. The American Journal of Sports Medicine; 22 (2): 167-70.
32. Granhed, J.; Morelli, B. (1988). Low back pain among retired wrestlers and heavyweight lifters. The American Journal of Sports Medicine; 16 (5): 530-3.
33. Beals, R.K.; Hickman N.W. (1972). Industrial injuries of the back and extremities. The Journal of Bone and Joint Surgery; 51 A (8): 1593-1611.

Chapter 4

1. Metropolitan Insurance Co. (1983). Metropolitan height and weight tables. Statistical Bulletin; 64 (January-June):2-9.
2. Willett, W.C.; et al. (1995). Weight, weight change, and coronary heart disease in women. Journal of the American Medical Association; 273 (6): 461-5.
3. Cook, A. (1994). Osteoporosis: Review and commentary. Journal of the Neuromusculoskeletal System; 2 (1): 9-18.
4. Raisz, L.G. (1988). Local and systemic factors in the pathogenesis of osteoporosis. The New England Journal of Medicine; 318 (14): 818-28.
5. American College of Sports Medicine, (1995). ACSM position stand on osteoporosis and exercise. Medicine and Science in Sports and Exercise; 27 (4): i-vii.
6. Yen, L.T.; et al. (1994). Corporate medical claim cost distributions and factors associated with high-cost status. Journal of Occupational Medicine; 36 (5): 505-15.

Chapter 5

1. Nachemson, A.L. (1983). Work for all. Clinical Orthopedics; 179: 77-85.
2. Hall, H.; Hadler, N.M. (1995). Controversy: low back school, education or exercise? Spine; 20 (9): 1097-8.
3. National Institute for Occupational Safety and Health (1981). Work practices guide for manual lifting. Cincinnati OH.: U.S. Department of Health and Human Services; NIOSH technical report No. 81-122.

4. Snook, S.H. (1987). Approaches to the control of back pain in industry: Job design, job placement and educational training. Spine; State of Art Review; 2 (1): 45-59.
5. Derebery, V.J.; et al. (1983). Delayed recovery in the patient with a work compensable injury. Journal of Occupational Medicine; 25 (11): 829-35.
6. Dwyer, A.P. (1987). Backache and its prevention. Clinical Orthopaedics and Related Research; 222: 35-43.
7. Editorial (1995). Weight control and exercise cardinal features of successful preventive gerontology. Journal of the American Medical Association; 274 (24): 1964-5.
8. Sandivk, L.; et al. (1993). Physical fitness as a predictor of mortality among healthy, middle-aged Norwegian men. New England Journal of Medicine; 328 (8): 533-7.
9. Paffenbarger, Jr. R.S.; et al. (1993). The association of changes in physical-activity level and other lifestyle characteristics with morality among men. New England Journal of Medicine; 328 (8): 538-45.
10. Paffenbarger, Jr. R.S.; et al. (1986). Physical activity, all-cause mortality, and longevity of college alumni. New England Journal of Medicine; 314 (10): 605-13.
11. Harris, S.S.; et al. (1989). Physical activity counseling for healthy adults as a primary preventive intervention in the clinical setting. Journal of the American Medical Association; 261 (24): 3590-8.
12. Rosenfield, O.; et al. (1989). The effect of physical training on objective and subjective measures of productivity and efficiency in industry. Ergonomics; 32 (8): 1019-28.
13. Beals, R.K.; Hickman, N.W. (1972). Industrial injuries of the back and extremities. The Journal of Bone and Joint Surgery; 51A (8): 1593.
14. Fordyce, W.E.; et al. (1981). Pain complaint-exercise performance in chronic pain. Pain; 10: 311-21.
15. Puig, M.M.; et al. (1982). Endorphin levels in cerebrospinal fluid of patients with postoperative and chronic pain. Anesthesiology; 57 (1): 1-4.
16. Shuy, B.C.; et al. (1982). Endorphin-medicated increase in pain threshold induced by long-lasting exercise in rates. Life Science; 30 (10): 833-40.

17. Colt, E.W.D.; Wardlaw, S.L.; Franz, A.G. (1981). The effect of running on plasma B-endorphin. Life Sciences; 28 (14): 1637-40.
18. Oyama, T.; Yamaya, R. (1980). Profound analgesic effects of B-endorphin in man. Lancet; 1: 122-4.
19. Linton, S.J. (1985). The relationship between activity and chronic pain. Pain; 21: 289-94.
20. International Society of Sport Psychology (1992). Physical activity and psychological benefits. The Physician and Sportsmedicine; 20 (10): 179-84.
21. Petruzzello, S.J.; et al. (1991). A meta-analysis on the anxiety-reducing effects of acute and chronic exercise. Outcomes and mechanisms. Sports Medicine; 11 (3): 143-82.
22. Devries, H.A.; et al. (1982). Fusimotor system involvement in the tranquilizer effect of exercise. American Journal of Physical Medicine; 61 (3): 111-22.
23. Berger, B.G.; Owen, D.R. (1983). Mood alteration with swimming—Swimmers really do "feel better." Psychosomatic Medicine; 45 (5): 425-33.
24. Hazard, R.C.; et al. (1989). Functional restoration with behavioral support: A one year prospective study of patients with chronic low-back pain. Spine; 14 (2): 157-61.
25. Snook, S.H.; et al. (1978). A study of three preventive approaches to low back injury. Journal of Occupational Medicine; 20: 478-81.

Chapter 7

1. Safran, M.R.; et al. (1988). The role of warm-up in muscular injury prevention. The American Journal of Sports Medicine; 16 (2): 123-7.
2. Wathen, D. (1987). Flexibility: Its place in warm-up activities. National Strength and Conditioning Association Journal; 9 (5): 26-7.
3. Chang, D.E.; et al. (1988). Limited joint mobility in power lifters. The American Journal of Sports Medicine; 16 (3): 280-4.
4. Chandler, J.T.; et al. (1990). Flexibility comparisons of junior elite tennis players to other athletes. The American Journal of Sports Medicine; 18 (2): 134-6.

5. Janda, V. (1978). Muscles, central nervous motor regulation and back problems. The Neurobiologic Mechanisms in Manipulative Therapy; edited by I.M. Korr, Plenum Press; pp. 27-41.
6. Lewit, K. (1985). Manipulative therapy in rehabilitation of the motor system. Butterworths; pp. 29-33.
7. Dorland's medical dictionary. 25th ed. (1974). Sherrington's law: When a muscle receives a nerve impulse to contract, its antagonist receives simultaneously an impulse to relax. p. 842.
8. American College of Sports Medicine (1991). Guidelines for exercise testing and prescription, 4th edition. Philadelphia: Lea & Febiger; p. 111.
9. Glick, S.M. (1980). Muscle strains: Prevention and treatment. The Physician and Sportsmedicine; 8 (11): 73-7.
10. Smith, L.L; et al. (1993). The effects of static and ballistic stretching on delayed onset muscle soreness and creative kinase. Research Quarterly for Exercise and Sport; 64 (1): 103-77.
11. Solveborn, S. (1985). The book about stretching. Tokyo and New York: Japan Publications Inc.; pp. 30, 31, 40, 41, 48, 57, 58, 62, 70, 74, 76.
12. White, A.H. (1983). Back school and other conservative approaches to low back pain. St. Louis: C.V. Mosby; p. 89.
13. Anderson, B. (1980) Stretching. Bolinas, Calif.: Shelter Publications; pp. 41, 59, 73, 84.
14 Uran, P. (1980). The complete stretching book. Mountain View, Calif.: Anderson World, Inc.; pp. 23-4.
15. Yang, P.J.; et al. (1985). Rotational vertebral artery occlusion at C1-C2. American Journal of Neurology and Rehabilation; 6: 98-100.
16. Josien, E. (1992). Extracranial vertebral artery dissection: nine-cases. Journal of Neurology; 239 (6): 327-30.
17. Pryse-Phillips, W. (1989). Infarction of the medulla and cervical cord after fitness exercise. Stroke; 30 (2): 292-94.
18. Leys, D.; et al. (1987). Bilateral spontaneous dissection of extracranial vertebral arteries. Journal of Neurology; 234 (4): 237-40.
19. Hanus, S.H.; et al. (1977). Vertebral artery occlusion complicating yoga exercises. Archives of Neurology; 34: 574-75.
20. Weintraub, M. (1993). Beauty parlor stroke syndrome: a report of 5 cases. Journal of the American Medical Association; 269 (16): 2085-6.

21. Sherman, D.G.; et al. (1981). Abrupt changes in head position and cerebral infarction. Stroke; 12: 2-6.

22. Gutowski, N.J.; et al. (1992). Unilateral upper cervical posterior spinal artery syndrome following sneezing. Journal Neuro Neurosurg Psychiatry; 55: 841-3.

23. Herr, R.D.; et al. (1992). Vertebral artery dissection from neck flexion during paroxysmal coughing. Annuals of Emergency Medicine; 21 (1): 88-91.

24. Buroker, K.C.; Schwane, J.A. (1989). Does post exercise static stretching alleviate delayed muscle soreness? The Physician and Sportsmedicine; 17 (6): 65-83.

25. Jorgensson, A. (1993). The iliopsoas muscle and the lumbar spine. Australian Journal of Physiotherapy; 39: 125-32.

Chapter 8

1. Metropolitan Insurance Co.(1983). Metropolitan height and weight tables. Statistical Bulletin; 64 (January-June): 2-9.

2. Willett, W.C.; et al. (1995). Weight, weight change, and coronary heart disease in women. Journal of the American Medical Association; 273 (6): 461-5.

3. Thygerson, A.L. (1989). Fitness and health. Boston: Jones and Bartlett Publishers; p. 200.

4. Johnson, L. (1985). The universal fitness institute, body fat. Cedar Rapids, Iowa: Universal Gym Co.

5. Kasch, F.W.; et al. (1990). The effect of physical activity and inactivity on aerobic power in older men. The Physician and Sportsmedicine; 18 (4): 73-83.

6. Jackson, A.S.; et al. (1995). Changes in aerobic power of men, ages 25-70 yr.. Medicine & Science in Sports & Exercise; 27 (1): 113-20.

7. Simopoulos, A.P. (1989). Nutrition and fitness. Journal of the American Medical Association; 261 (19): 2862-3.

8. Lee, I.M.; et al. (1993). Body weight and mortality. Journal of the American Medical Association; 270 (23): 2823-8.

9. Bicycling Magazine. (1992). Counting calories: August; 16.

10. American Dietetic Association (1987). Position of the American Dietetic Association: Nutrition for Physical Fitness, and Athletic Per-

formance for Adults. Journal of the American Dietetic Association; 87: 933-9.

11. Wood, P.D. (1993). Impact of experimental manipulation of energy intake and expenditure on body composition. Critical Reviews in Food Science and Nutrition; 33 (4/5): 369-73.
12. Wood, P.D.; et al. (1988). Changes in plasma lipids and lipoprotein in overweight men during weight loss through dieting as compared with exercise. The New England Journal of Medicine; 319 (18): 1173-9.
13. Work, J.A. (1990). Exercise for the overweight patient. The Physician and Sportsmedicine; 18 (7): 113-22.
14. Cook, A. (1994). Osteoporosis: Review and commentary. Journal of the Neuromusculoskeletal System; 2 (1): 9-18.
15. The American College of Sports Medicine (1990). The recommended quantity and quality of exercise for developing and maintaining cardiorespiratory and muscular fitness in healthy adults. Medicine and Science in Sports and Exercise; 22 (2): 265-74.
16. Tucci, J.J. (1988). A study of urban bicycling accidents. The American Journal of Sports Medicine; 16 (2): 181-4.
17. McLennan, J.G.; et al. (1988). Accident prevention in competitive cycling. The American Journal of Sports Medicine; 16 (3): 266-8.
18. Koszuta, L.E. (1989). From sweats to swimsuits: Is water exercise the wave of the future? The Physician and Sportsmedicine; 17 (4): 203-6.
19. Ekstrand, J.; Gillquist, J. (1982). The frequency of muscle tightness and injuries in soccer players. The American Journal Of Sports Medicine; 10 (2): 75-8.
20. Kurosawa, H.; et al. (1991). Radiographic findings of degeneration in cervical spines of middle-aged soccer players. Skeletal Radiology; 20 (6): 437-40.
21. Weir, M.R.; Smith, D.S. (1989). Stress reaction of the pars interarticularis leading to spondylolysis. A cause of adolescent low back pain. Journal of Adolescent Health Care; 10 (6): 573-7.
22. Herskowitz, A.; Selesnick, H. (1993). Back injuries in basketball players. Clinics in Sports Medicine; 12 (2): 293-306.
23. Wheeler, L.P. (1987). Common musculoskeletal dance injuries. Chiropractic Sports Medicine; 1 (1): 17-23.
24. Koszuta, L.E. (1986). Low-impact aerobics: Better than traditional aerobic dance? The Physician and Sportsmedicine; 14 (7): 156-61.

25. Garrick, J.G.; et al. (1986). The epidemiology of aerobic dance injuries. American Journal of Sports Medicine; 14 (1): 67-72.

26. Cooper, P.G.; ed. (1988). Aerobics: Theory & practice. Sherman Oaks, Calif.: The Aerobics and Fitness Association of America; pp. 143-56.

Chapter 9

1. The American College of Sports Medicine (1990). The recommended quantity and quality of exercise for developing and maintaining cardiorespiratory and muscular fitness in healthy adults. Medicine and Science in Sports and Exercise; 22(2): 265-74.
2. The American College of Sports Medicine (1991). Guidelines for exercise testing and prescription, 4th edition. Philadelphia: Lea & Febiger; pp. 93-110.
3. Harris, S.S.; et al. (1989). Physical activity counseling for healthy adults as a primary preventive intervention in the clinical setting. Journal of the American Medical Association; 261 (24): 3590-8.
4. Fox, E.L.; Mathews, D.K. (1981). The physiological basis of physical education and athletics. Philadelphia: Saunders College Publishing; pp. 262-6.
5. Borg, G. (1982). Psychophysical bases of perceived exertion. Medicine and Science in Sports and Exercise: 14 (5); 377-81.
6. Drake, G. (1992). Coach's corner. Bicycling Magazine: April; 81-5.

Chapter 10

1. Fiatarone, M.A.; et al. (1990). High-intensity strength training in nonagenarians: Effects on skeletal muscle. Journal of the American Medical Association; 263 (22): 3029-34.
2. Frontera, W.R.; et al. (1988). Strength conditioning in older men: Skeletal muscle hypertrophy and improved function. Journal of Applied Physiology; 64: 1038-44.
3. Larsson, L.; et al. (1979). Muscle strength and speed of movement in relation to age and muscle morphology. Journal of Applied Physiology; 46 (3): 451-6.
4. Thorstensson, A. (1977). Observation on strength training and detraining. Acta Physicolgica Scandinavica; 100: 491-3.

5. Cureton, K.J.; et al. (1986). Exercise-induced muscle hypertrophy in men and women. Medicine and Science in Sports and Exercise; 18 (suppl): S77.
6. Thorstensson, A.; et al. (1976). Effects in strength training on enzyme activities and fibre characteristics in human skeletal muscle. Acta Physiologica Scandinvica; 96: 392-8.
7. Nelson, M.E.; et al. (1994). Effects of high-intensity strength training on multiple risk factors for osteoporotic fractures. Journal of the American Medical Association; 272 (24): 1909-14.
8. Stacey, R.A. (1989). Osteoporosis: Exercise therapy, pre- and post diagnosis. Journal of Manipulative and Physiological Therapeutics; 12 (3): 211-19.
9. Sinaki, M.; et al. (1986). Relationship between bone mineral density of spine and strength of back extensors in healthy postmenopausal women. Mayo Clinic Proceedings; 61: 116-22.
10. Sianki, M.; et al. (1974). Bone mineral content: Relationship to muscle strength in normal subjects. Archive of Physical Medicine and Rehabilitation; 55: 508-12.
11. Nevitt, M.C.; et al. (1989). Risk factors for recurrent falls: A prospective study. Journal of the American Medical Association; 261 (18): 2663-8.
12. Work, J.A. (1989). Strength training: A bridge to independence for the elderly. The Physician and Sportsmedicine; 17 (11): 134-40.
13. Coaches Roundtable (1987). Breathing during weight training. National Strength and Conditioning Association Journal; 9 (5): 17-25.
14. Harman, E.A.; et al. (1989). Effects of a belt on intra-abdominal pressure during weight lifting. Medicine and Science in Sports and Exercise; 21 (2): 186-90.
15. Harman, E. (1994). Weight training safety: A biomechanical perspective. Strength and Conditioning Journal; October; 55-60.
16. Hamill, B.P. (1994). Relative safety of weightlifting and weight training. Journal of Strength and Conditioning Research; 8 (1): 53-7.
17. Coaches Roundtable (1983). Prevention of athletic injuries through strength training and conditioning. National Strength and Conditioning Association Journal; April-May; 14-19.

18. Sinaki, M.; Mikkelsen, B.A. (1984). Postmenopausal osteoporosis: Flexion versus extension exercises. Archives of Physical Medicine and Rehabilitation; 65: 593-6.
19. Berg, H.E.; et al. (1994). Dynamic neck strength training on pain and function. Archives of Physical Medicine and Rehabilitation; 75: 661-5.
20. Fahey, T.D. (1989). Basic weight training. Mountain View, Calif.: Mayfield Publishing Company.
21. O'Connor, B.; Simmons, J.; O'Shea, P. (1989). Weight training today. St. Paul: West Publishing Co.

Chapter 11

1. Martens, R. (1987). Coaches guide to sport psychology. Champaign Ill.: Human Kinetics Publishers, Inc.
2. Roberts, G.C., ed. (1992). Motivation in sport and exercise. Champaign Ill.: Human Kinetics Publishers, Inc.
3. Rejeski, W.J.; Kenney, E.A. (1988). Fitness motivation: Preventing participant dropout. Champaign Ill.: Life Enhancement Publications.
4. Orlick, T. (1986). Psyching for sport: mental training for athletes. Champaign, Ill.: Leisure Press.
5. Harris, S.S.; et al. (1989). Physical activity counseling for healthy adults as a primary preventive intervention in the clinical setting. Journal of the American Medical Association; 261 (24): 3590-8.

Index

About the Author

WILL WHITNEY has been a practicing chiropractor for fifteen years and a collegiate physical education instructor for seven years. He is a state-appointed medical evaluator for on-the-job injuries and disabilities and has postdoctorate training in occupational health. In addition, Dr. Whitney has served as a chiropractic consultant for the South Korean Olympic boxing team and as a team doctor for numerous amateur athletic organizations. He served a six-year term as an appointed member of the California Chiropractic Association's ethics committee.

Dr. Whitney earned a graduate degree and teaching credential in Health, Physical Education, and Recreation. His master's thesis researched the different preventive approaches to back pain within the workplace. Dr. Whitney has served as an advisory board member to the Contra Costa County Department of Health Services Prevention Program. His project for the program has prompted individuals to follow a healthier and active lifestyle through community-based activities.

Dr. Whitney is married and has two children. He currently is a member of the American College of Sports Medicine and regularly exercises the back-friendly way. Although he trains on a stationary bike, he has completed numerous bicycle century (100-mile or 100-kilometer) rides. He also enjoys walking the countryside trails of his native California.